With best wishes – and thanks
for kindness shown – to Deirdre

Michael

THE VITAL SPARK!

THE VITAL SPARK!

Fitting In With Epilepsy

MICHAEL IGOE

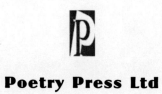

Poetry Press Ltd

THE VITAL SPARK!

MICHAEL IGOE

First Published in 2008 by

Poetry Press Ltd
26 Park Grove, Edgware, Middx, HA8 7SJ

ISBN 9780954859688

CONTENTS

ACKNOWLEDGEMENTS

For many years, I have had the ambition to write about the personal experience of epilepsy, but have been unable every time before now to complete more than an opening page or two, only then to lose heart and abandon the project. As the content of this book will demonstrate, the dragging up of painful memories has been too much to tolerate. Then my conscience would strike again, with the same result. And then again, and then again.

I owe it to Mrs Judy Karbritz and her gentle encouragement that I have finally managed to complete the work, with huge relief. Her contribution to the text, wisely, was nothing whatever. Instead, as each section was e-mailed to her, she provided some critical comment, but no more than this.

I've said 'wisely' since there's no-one who can really comment on the experience of any form of disability except the disabled person himself. This applies as much to neurological conditions as to any other – perhaps even more. There are many well-meaning people who comment on medical conditions with no possible awareness of the inner truth as it affects the disabled person. They see, but they can't feel.

This general truth, perhaps, applies rather more to epilepsy than to many other conditions. For practically all of recorded history, epilepsy, probably the commonest of neurological conditions, has been plagued by an association with superstition. There's possible evidence that this notion actually predates

3

known history. In many parts of the world, traces – sometimes more than traces - of this idea remain, even in what we fondly imagine are 'developed' countries. A lingering concept like this, spoken or not, makes epilepsy, in many instances, more of a social than a medical difficulty. It's largely for this reason, I'm convinced, that the real numbers of people with epilepsy aren't generally realised: worldwide perhaps forty million or so, many or most remaining unmedicated.

My thanks go to Mrs Mary Anderson (Maggie Blue) for her imaginative artwork used in the cover of this work, and to George Raybould of New York. During my voluntary contribution of material to his now discontinued web site for people with epilepsy, it was George who helped me ease my style into a far less formal one than I tended to write in until then.

It goes almost without saying that I must acknowledge the efforts of the various medical staff over many years to help me with this apparently intractable condition. These range from the neurologists of the Southern General Hospital, Glasgow, to the staff of the University Hospital of North Durham. Nor should we forget the indispensable paramedics and general practitioners.

This book is dedicated, however, perhaps most of all to my ever-caring and supportive family.

Michael Igoe   Durham, UK. May 2008

AUTHOR'S FOREWORD

At the risk of perhaps repeating some points made in the text of the work which follows, it's important to make certain important facts clear. First, I've tried to give a picture of some aspects of the social, personal and other features of life with epilepsy, at least as I've experienced it. I hope and believe that some of what I've written will chime with the experiences of others with this still little mentioned and strangely neglected condition and those close to them. Too often, even now, people with epilepsy are left to feel isolated and alone when there's no reason that they should be.

What this isn't - and this point must be stressed - is any sort of guidebook to the medical aspects of the condition. These are something which only a qualified medical expert can advise on, and I most certainly don't fall into that category. I'm a lay person with many years' experience of the condition, much of it written down soon after onset of attacks, and can speak about it only from that point of view. I make a point of passing copies of this material to my epilepsy nurse and the consultant who deals with my case, in the hope of providing valuable information.

There are some mistaken ideas in particular which surround epilepsy which I'd like to deal with here. The first is that it's essentially a children's condition, and that the young person may be confidently expected to 'grow out of it' in time, almost like teenage acne. This may happen - it was hoped for in my own case long ago - but certainly isn't always what actually does happen. I developed epilepsy, for no apparent reason, in my adolescent years. Regrettably, it has stayed with me and I've simply learned to live with it in the more than forty years since then. It's never stood in my way, for I haven't allowed it to, except when there was obvious danger involved in my intentions. Then, but only then, I've reconsidered. However, I've never found too much caution at all preferable to too little. The middle way has always been best.

Another instance of the condition appearing outside childhood is my late father, who developed epilepsy in his mid-sixties as a result of a stroke. Epilepsy late in life, although not at all unusual, is barely mentioned, unless in some other connection. Infantile convulsions are relatively common in young children, but only on occasion, as I understand it, are signs of epilepsy. An expert's advice should always be asked even so, just to make sure.

Strangely, my own experience of the condition was actually an advantage after this development in my father. I was able to reassure family members that, despite alarming appearances, his fits caused him no pain. There might be a headache after the seizure, but nothing worse. Or there might sometimes be some incontinence. However, both features applied to me too, and they caused me only occasional problems. I'm not convinced they quite believed what I had to say. I can only hope so. Do they quite believe what I have to say about my own seizures? I can only do my best.

Another notion which is gaining ground if anything is that epilepsy is more a woman's condition than a man's. There's little evidence for this.

6

Pregnancy, for example, can result in fewer seizures or perhaps more, or perhaps make no difference at all. What does matter is to keep in contact with a doctor, who can keep a check on the level of anti-seizure medication in the body. I have a suspicion that this idea, that women are more likely to develop epilepsy than men, has a great deal to do with men's traditional unwillingness to ask for medical advice. It's almost as if illness were somehow thought unmanly. In some cases, of course, with a number of conditions, help is asked for only when it's tragically too late for much to be done.

It's partly for this reason, and partly for simple convenience, that I haven't used terms like 'he/she' etc in this book, unless it was absolutely necessary. 'He' and 'his' etc should be taken to apply as much to women as to men.

And it's largely for the same reason, of convenience, that I've used the terms 'seizure', 'attack', 'fit' and 'onset' as more or less interchangeable. If there actually is a difference, it would need a specialist to identify them. As far as the person experiencing the attack is concerned, almost certainly without a specialist close by, in most cases such distinctions count for little or nothing at the time.

I've deliberately subtitled this book *Fitting In With Epilepsy* to stress that the condition, however it's sometimes represented or thought of, isn't some sort of death sentence. It needn't get in the way of what you really want to accomplish, including living a normal, productive life, just so long as you're determined to do so and to ignore the prophets of misery that I can almost guarantee will appear in your life. Some of these mean well, certainly, and these you should gently, but very firmly, ignore. Then there the others, those determined to save you from yourself. Almost invariably, these rely on hopelessly outdated, inaccurate information. These it makes sense to ignore completely. You, the person with epilepsy, know what it involves, far more than any of them possibly can.

To explain my own position: I was diagnosed with epilepsy in my mid-teens, now four decades ago. I wasn't greatly shaken at first; more, if anything, by the medication then available than by the condition itself. That's only natural, for it's commonly difficult to get used to powerful medication acting directly on the brain.

Except where other people have interfered, having epilepsy has done nothing to prevent me from getting on with an accomplished life. I'm a college graduate three times over with a range of awards for work in languages, which fascinate me and I know always will. I've worked as a teacher, a translator and occasionally as an interpreter. I'm widely travelled, which has made full use of my language skills. Along the way, I've gained a whole range of practical qualifications besides.

And that's one reason for the title of this book, *The Vital Spark*. 'Vital', as far as I'm concerned, means 'life-giving'. It may sound almost illogical to say this, but it's perfectly true: I don't think I could have managed in life quite so well without having epilepsy. It's given me that extra push to fight against the odds and to confront sometimes bigoted people who have tried to belittle me. My weapons of choice weren't aggression or bitterness, but clear-headed assertiveness and my awareness of having a finer record of achievement than most of my critics. In a generally able-bodied world, it's essential for any disabled person to develop an extra level of self-belief.

It's true to say that I haven't always won and the road behind me has a list of casualties, some in particular that, even after many years, continue to sadden me. However, I believe I can chalk up more successes than failures, and there are other casualties on that same road who will now know better than to mock epilepsy or 'epileptics', as if somehow inferior beings, without expecting a reply – at least from me. For it's true to say that epilepsy, for most people with it, is more a social than a medical problem. Whatever the reason for this attitude, society feels uneasy with epilepsy.

I'll pull no punches and be quite blunt about it: epilepsy can be vicious, often hitting for no obvious reason. It can leave you injured, sometimes badly, as it has done occasionally with me. All you can do then is tackle it over time, learn to live with it, and emerge stronger for the experience. This isn't just pep talk from some well-meaning individual. At times, I've found myself on the verge of near-total despair, at one time scarcely able to walk or even speak, a grim prospect for a linguist and traveller. However, I surmounted them and came out the winner.

A point well worth making, however, is that often it's not been the condition itself that caused the sense of despair. It was far more the attitudes of many people to it and, because of it, to me. These included, painfully often, people who hadn't so much as seen epilepsy, but only imagined what it must be like and that I must, strangely, be some sort of threat to them because of it. It's nonsensical and irrational attitudes like these which, as a rule, cause people with epilepsy most of the difficulties of their condition. This point can't be stressed strongly enough, for these attitudes are the cause of much discrimination and needless strains and unhappiness for both those with the condition and their families. It's time for someone with the condition (I refuse to speak of myself as a 'sufferer') to put the record straight.

TO MICHAEL

I met Michael Igoe through the Internet several years ago and we have become firm friends.

I recently co-wrote a book about Obsessive Compulsive Disorder with a friend who suffers from OCD as we felt that although many eminent doctors have written about this condition, it would be helpful to read about it from the point of view of someone who daily lives with the obsessions that rule how she even walks and bathes and also control her thoughts.

We had extremely positive feedback from the OCD book and it set my mind to thinking that a book about epilepsy should be written from a similar point of view. And who else by, but my friend Michael?

I have long respected Michael's ability to write with a light touch about serious subjects and I set about bullying him to write about his life with epilepsy as I believe it will familiarize people like me who would never consider reading a textbook on epilepsy but are always interested in stories and the people behind them.

Michael has emailed me chapter by chapter and I admit to continually urging him forward as I have wanted to read the next instalment.

And now it's here. From reading it I have discovered so much about epilepsy but more importantly, I have been privileged to learn about the life of my friend Michael Igoe.

Judy Karbritz
London, 2008

I SIPPED ESPRESSO

I sipped espresso in a bar
Half-eaten sandwich, toasted cheese
A girl strummed on an old guitar
Until an aura of unease

It felt like movies where new scenes
Lack continuity and sense
All logic flies, and nothing means
The same, the world's locked in pretence

My eyes unclosed, strange voices droned
One man concerned, the rest disgusted
"Is he drunk?" "He must be stoned"
"Quick, call the police, let's get him busted!"

A voice asked, "Has he had a fit
Or do you think he's just a nutter?"
I tried to speak, to move, to sit
As I lay there, in the gutter

13

1: FITS AND STARTS

A quiet uproar, if such a thing is possible, in the semi-darkness. Why wasn't I just being left to sleep? I was so tired, so hideously tired, I didn't care what was happening. I was wrung out, exhausted.

So many weird things. Ranged along the bedroom wall, just opposite, in the faint light of a partly-opened door stood my family, eyes wide and staring, as if they were facing a firing squad at the very moment that the safety catches are clicked off. And just above me, another face, this one unfamiliar, staring down anxiously and muttering. After a moment or two, this new person stood up and went over to my family, speaking quietly. Whatever he said, it seemed to give them little comfort. Finally the door closed again, and I sank back thankfully into darkness. Whatever had happened, it didn't matter any longer. It was over.

It was a bright November morning when I was wakened, but only just still morning. My parents, normally sticklers for timekeeping, had left me asleep until well past 11 am. There was to be no school that day, I was told, perhaps not for a day or two more. There was a sense that something was in the air, something I couldn't identify. Some arrangements would have to be made that I didn't question. Still, it was an unexpected holiday, so why should I ask any questions? What was plain was that I wasn't in any

15

trouble, something that would have concerned me. But still there was that strange something in the atmosphere, something I'd never felt before. And what had happened during that night, with the turmoil in my bedroom? Probably, I eventually decided, it was just a particularly vivid dream, however unlikely that seemed. I just put it out of my thoughts and said no more.

Then, after a few days, arrived a franked brown envelope, inviting me to the Neurology Department of a nearby hospital. I was to come along with a responsible adult. Neurology? What was that? To a fourteen-year-old like me, the word meant nothing at all. The dictionary definition was little, if any, help, and left me even more confused than ever. It was just too complicated.

The day came, and we left, my mother and I, in good time. No point in asking questions on the way, I reasoned, for I'd find out soon enough when we reached our destination. Anyway, little was said on the journey. That strange, indefinable something hung over us both, even yet. In actual fact, I'd already given up the comforting notion that I'd simply been dreaming that night. Something very real had happened. But the mystery remained unanswered – what had it been?

The local hospital, about seven miles away, was a forbidding place. Once of red sandstone, it was now heavily blackened by the city's industry. Somehow, I seemed to realise even then, that seemed appropriate. We were ushered into a grim waiting room and left there for some time. Then came my turn to take part in a bizarre ritual.

16

My head was covered in glue and electrodes were attached. I was instructed to lie on a table and given a long series of mysterious instructions. I was to lift this leg, now that, eyes closed, then open. The same with my arms: lift one, then the other, eyes closed or open as I was told to do. Just what was going on?

At the far end of the bed, just beyond hearing, stood two white-coated medical staff, who knowingly whispered to one another and nodded gravely as a long roll of paper passed through a machine, attached to a hopelessly complex array of dials and gauges, just before them.

An hour or so later, it was all over and I could return home to wash the glue from my hair, as I was longing to do. As I walked by, however, towards the exit, I couldn't stop myself from stealing a glance at the machine behind me. Here and there on the long paper roll, protruding from an otherwise generally straight line, were some high, pointed marks. I didn't realise then that these were the signs of characteristic irregularities or sparks in my brain electricity, the 'spikes' that indicated epilepsy. In another sense, they represented the mountains that I would have to climb in my future life.

So far from a dream that night, I later discovered, my brother had noticed me strangely writhing in my sleep, close to choking, and the unfamiliar face had been that of the emergency doctor, called out before dawn. It was easily possible that, if my brother by pure good luck, hadn't been temporarily sharing my bedroom, I wouldn't have survived till the morning.

No great time later, my mother, in a carefully staged offhand manner, asked how I'd feel if I were told I had epilepsy. Epilepsy? The term was at least as vague as neurology. All I knew was that it was some sort of medical condition, one rarely mentioned. For that reason alone, surely it could hardly be anything much to be concerned about.

It didn't take long to give a light-hearted reply. It might just make me special, I commented, someone separate. In later years, these were to prove highly prophetic words.

2: COMING OF AGE

My unexpected holiday wasn't to last long. Within days, I was back at school, with only one minor change. I had a small bottle of medication to be carried with me at all times. Occasionally I noticed, during lessons I'd have unintended daydreams. Still, to a frequent daydreamer like me, these scarcely mattered, though I did find them puzzling.

It was only a year or two until certificate examinations, and I was determined to do well, especially in the area that fascinated me: ancient languages and history. This meant hours of homework. From time to time, however, I found myself earnestly warned by my family not to overdo things. I ignored these warnings, defiance which occasionally caused some minor friction.

When the time came, I did do well and went early to university, to follow a deliberately demanding, four-year course, again in ancient languages and history. This meant even more work to bring home in the evenings. And it meant, too, even more warnings to be ignored. If this was what I wanted to do and obviously had to do, I wondered, why were my family so concerned? It made no sense.

One of the demands made of any language student at the time was that he must be prepared to

19

spend some time in the country where the chosen language was spoken, so as to gain some feeling for the culture and background. This was the way in which I discovered the wonders of overseas travel, which I still enjoy, epilepsy or not. At the time, in the mid-1960s, air travel was still beyond the reach of most people, especially students. That first journey meant four days' travel by train through a series of different countries, each with its different language and ways. Certainly it was demanding, but well worth my effort.

Most of those countries I've visited again since, after that original taster. There were the mountains of Austria, for example, and the breathtaking and shocking sight of Skopje, capital of Macedonia, still recovering from a major earthquake not long before. The main railway station showed a massive split down the front, its public clock stopped at the time of the disaster. This, I realised, was how the world could really be. It wasn't at all an extension of the comfortable background from which I'd come. Without realising it at the time, I was now genuinely growing up.

At last the train ended its journey, at Larissa in central Athens. A tight fist seemed to grip my entrails, that sense of unease that everyone knows when faced with the unfamiliar. What was I now about to see, and have to cope with for myself, aged seventeen and as far from home as I could be while still in Europe?

I discovered within minutes that it was turmoil, a stunning uproar of voices, babbling, babbling in all directions. What were these people saying? I should know, but I didn't. It's what every linguist encounters: the contrast between language as read in a book and as he first hears it spoken in the street.

I was totally lost, standing there in the burning sun of early June. We stumbled, a fellow-student and I, to a nearby street café and, thankfully, found seats there to rest on and take stock of our bewilderment. How could anyone live in such a noisy, turbulent place? Everywhere, the people, seated and standing, seemed to be squabbling and arguing at as high a volume as I could imagine possible.

A heavily built waiter appeared and barked something which was obviously a demand for our order. We pointed at something which was scrawled on the menu, evidently coffee. And our first meal on arrival was a single piece of what I've since found out is matzo bread. It was fitting, in a way, to have an almost biblical welcome (at a price, but very little, in strange little aluminium coins) to such an ancient city.

The sun was sinking, strangely early as I thought then, used only to the North, in a violet-tinted twilight, as we crept wearily to the grubby lodgings that had been pre-arranged, not far from the city centre. It had been a shock to encounter strange places and strange ways at first hand, rather than through a train window, but a healthy shock. Now rest was very much needed – but less from the journey itself than the experience of arrival.

The next days, one after another, were just a repetition of the first: a torrent of unintelligible

21

babbling in blazing sunlight. But, only very slowly, I began to realise that street signs and the posters haphazardly plastered on almost any vacant spot had just a little meaning that I could recognise, then a little more, almost by the day. My spirits began to lift. But those voices remained impenetrable. Why so fast and why so loud? Why couldn't I even begin to understand what they were saying? At one level, it was horrifying, and at another, captivating. This was simply this people's way, and it probably always had been.

I think it was after about ten days or so, that what had seemed impossible at first suddenly happened. I was at a café table near the main market, feeling something between elation and despair. With only a small amount of my coffee drunk, I realised something incredible. Without so much as noticing it at first, I had been following the drift of an argument (of course – in this strange country it seemed it could be nothing else) between two elderly men sitting at a nearby table. The shock was so stunning it was almost physical and knocked me from my seat, sending my coffee flying.

I'd finally experienced what the Germans refer to as *Sprachgefühl* (there appears to be no English word for it). It's the feeling of or for a language when it, so to speak, enters your bloodstream. Embarrassing, I thought, even then, that the people who helped me back to my feet were the two men I had unintentionally been eavesdropping on. I said nothing about it, only thanked them for their help. The waiter pretended not to notice, but just replaced my coffee. Had he guessed what had just happened? I still suspect so. And the two men recommenced their argument.

As time passed, my understanding of these people, so strange at first, grew. No, they weren't at all separated from the history and the old mythology I knew. These could have come from only here. The places I knew from myths and legends, one after another, I discovered truly did exist; were genuine. It simply didn't matter if I so often had to travel in impossibly ancient, crowded buses to trudge around in intensely hot, pine-scented dust, far out in the countryside, to see them and feel their atmosphere for myself.

Impression after impression, day after day, but not all for the good, or perhaps, for me at least, they were. There was another side, I discovered, to life here, just like anywhere else. I came across desperate poverty, and elderly people driven to insanity by their experiences in the Occupation of the 1940s, not so greatly long before. In a small country town, I found a rifle thrust in my face. I was assured, this was simply a case of mistaken identity.

There were civil uprisings in darkened city squares. There was the night I found myself, an eighty-year-old woman beside me, crouched behind an impossibly small overturned street café table, each of us desperately holding our breath for fear of discovery. If the riot police, whose boots we could see as they prowled here and there within arm's reach, so much as suspected that they had noticed either of us choking on the tear gas fumes filling the atmosphere, we knew what we could expect. They weren't noted for kindly ways or their understanding.

These characteristics weren't part of their remit. Yet wasn't this Goodwill Square, of all places? Such, however, is human life, I realised. It's so often an outright contradiction – and not just abroad. This was to be one of the most valuable lessons I ever learned.

It wasn't long after the grinding of armoured vehicles had died away that it seemed safe to return to my apartment, taking care to move along only the darker lanes. Shortly after I arrived back, still ill at ease and had finally gathered myself, word came that, lying in that very square, supposedly dedicated to friendly relations, was a young man only a year or two older than I was. He could never return to his home, unless carried by family or friends. He had been struck with the full violence of one of the tear gas shells fired into the crowd, only a short distance from where I had stood myself, however unintentionally. I had accidentally walked into a political demonstration which the authorities of the time had ruthlessly suppressed. He had very probably simply made the same mistake – at the cost of his life.

This, I realised, was the true meaning of tragedy. He had simply been in the wrong place. From then on, the inscriptions I read on monuments, of whatever age, carried a meaning that they had never had for me before.

Finally, it was time to leave this city and country of mayhem that had by now become part of me, probably for ever. As the train, almost like a magic carpet, sped across national boundaries, and advertising hoardings for the most familiar items changed from language to language, I found myself aware that the person now returning to his family could never again be the same as the one who had left all that time before. And for that entire period, strangely, whatever the sometimes extreme circumstances, I had never known a single onset of epilepsy.

I brought back with me vital lessons as I re-entered my family's home. One was that it isn't a society's duty to accommodate itself to an individual, but for the individual to accommodate himself to the society he comes across. Another was that a society will accept a person who is prepared to be part of it and contribute to it. That is, usually.

3: THE TRUTH STRIKES HOME

Then, on my return, it was back to the remainder of the course, just as before. Finally I emerged with a series of awards in language work. There could be no stopping me now. My one ambition had always been to work in education, for which I'd need to attend a one-year training course. I sent for the application form, filled it in as required and forwarded it back to the training college, confident of the result. I had done everything needed, and more besides.

On a bright August morning, the phone rang for me. It was the college medical staff, to inform me curtly that I needn't trouble to turn up on admissions day, for, with my medical condition, I wouldn't be accepted. With that, the phone was abruptly put down.

Even after so many years, I still vividly remember that call. In some strange way, the phone in my hand seemed more real than reality itself. My eyes fixed on its creamy-white colour and on every mark and whorl on its surface. I surely couldn't have heard those words. Had I imagined it? Yet I knew that I hadn't. Such things couldn't happen, surely, especially for some reason on such bright, warm days? But they could. I'd finally come face to face with my society's view of epilepsy, and that face wasn't a welcoming one. I'd been rejected on medical grounds, without as much as a medical examination.

I don't really know what happened afterwards, but my family tell me that I was clearly stunned, silent and withdrawn. I know that I went for long walks, but have no idea where. Only one clue suggests itself. I love the scent of pine trees, but their scent, strangely, both comforts me and makes me almost shudder, even now.

After some days, I began to regain myself. To be rejected in this way just didn't make the slightest sense. I went to a local doctor, long familiar with my history, for a personal inspection. He commented favourably on me: I should clearly be accepted now. His report on me formed part of my appeal. This, however, was rejected too. The training college simply had no place for a person with my condition. I was unacceptable. What I'd achieved in the past years just didn't count.

Despair developed into determination. It was possible at the time to teach without a certificate for a fixed period, and it was on this arrangement that I taught a range of subjects at a local school, without incidents. Yes, I knew, this was the career for me. At the end of that year I found a college which would accept me and gained a certificate with merit. I had proved who was in the right and began to teach again.

After a year or two an offer came my way, of a period as a research student in northern England. This was a prize not to be missed. I delightedly snapped it up. It was anything but easy going, involving long days, sometimes seven a week,

27

working well into the evening.　　However,　　my memory of it still is of a near-idyll. I was doing what interested me most. I advised on the mythological theme of a public sculpture. And it was here, too, that I met my now ex-wife.

Gradually, however, as the two years passed and the idyll was coming to an end, I knew that I had to return soon. What would I find, I wondered, when I went back, for there seemed to be no other choice? Surely things had improved, at least a little, I told myself. But it took some effort not to sense something sinister in the air.

The last day came, and it was time to return. My memory, as I left a place I had loved so much, was of someone playing a recording of Elgar's *Enigma Variations*. Somehow, that seemed so appropriate in the circumstances. Life with epilepsy, I now knew, was itself an enigma. It always had been in history, and largely still was.

It wasn't difficult, with my additional experience, to find a teaching position in my home area. Unlike before, however, I began to experience minor, flickering attacks. Each time this was seen happening, I was summoned to the headmaster's office and ordered to explain myself. Why wasn't I taking my medication? But I was, I replied, for only I would be the loser if I didn't. This question of his was ludicrous. It was as if he held me personally responsible for my health condition.

Very well, then, he demanded, if I was taking it, why were these attacks occurring? The perfect medication for my condition, I had to inform him, over and over, didn't yet exist. We'd long had aspirin, yet people still experienced persistent headaches, didn't they? Didn't I have a colleague who suffered from severe migraine? He had to admit the truth of this, but for some reason it was an argument which seemed to outrage him more than any other.

I've since realised the explanation for this odd difference. Migraine was a word, a notion, he was familiar with. Epilepsy, however, wasn't.

Had anyone complained about my standard of work, I asked? No, no-one had. Then what was the point of interrogating me in this way? The conclusion, I gradually realised, could only be that I – or more correctly my condition – for some reason made him feel insecure in some way. I could scarcely suggest this to him outright, obviously, but there could be no other reason for this repeated questioning and accusation.

Attitudes to epilepsy, I found to my cost, clearly hadn't changed. If anything, they'd hardened. And then again, there was the same questioning at the next onset, the same replies, and then yet again. I knew that I had to stay on my guard, which itself put extra strain on me and so often made onsets all the more likely.

Colleagues began to avoid me in the corridors. Some even muttered threats. This, naturally, meant still further caution, for I knew I couldn't look to them for help or support, very much the opposite. They were actually aggravating the difficulties to which they objected. But why treat me this way? How could I possibly be a threat to them? That was certainly the impression their behaviour left on me – that I was seen as some sort of danger. Slowly, only very unwillingly, I found memories returning of that night in Goodwill Square some years before. Those prowling security guards, that need to conceal myself from their attention. Only now, these were supposedly my work colleagues.

At the close of that year, I found myself faced with a final offer, or more correctly an ultimatum. I could resign, the headmaster told me, and count on a favourable reference, or be dismissed. I was still so very green then, unused to the ways of the world. Just before the beginning of the summer holiday, I handed him my resignation. At last we would be rid of each other. I could continue my career somewhere more tolerant. Surely nowhere else could be anything like this dreadful place.

It was only a few weeks later, not long after my marriage, that my parents arrived at our flat carrying a letter addressed to me at their home. It was formal notice that my licence to work in schools was withdrawn, in effect for life, the equivalent of a doctor's being struck off the register. I'd had no opportunity of representation, no warning even that my case was being considered. At the very beginning of married life, my key to a professional career had been snatched away. This was my supposedly favourable reference.

More than three decades later, this prohibition remains in force. Repeatedly, at the time, I appealed against the decision to disbar me, sometimes with highly placed support. It became obvious, however, that no-one had any intention of rethinking the matter. Without even trying to do so,

30

I'd made powerful enemies, simply on the basis of a minor medical condition. This was what had come of my efforts to gain my certificate and what I'd achieved with such effort earlier. In professional terms, I no longer existed. I was now a non-person.

Yet, even now, it wasn't all grim. In the weeks and months following, more letters for me arrived at my parents' address. They were from pupils I'd taught, expressing their support and thanks for my efforts. I treasure these even now. They count for more, as far as I'm concerned, than the letter announcing the withdrawal of my licence. They proved that there was such a thing as human kindness to set against official disapproval and heartlessness.

Incredibly, the most recent of these letters arrived at my present home more than thirty years after the event. Anything more heartening I can't imagine, and I've added this letter to my earlier collection. In the very teeth of what had been done, there was confirmation of my own view: whatever else I might be, it wasn't a failure or a *persona non grata*. And there were others who agreed.

From time to time, I find myself thinking back to schooldays, when I returned just after my first seizure (or seizures, for it's possible there were more than one which went unnoticed). It's well known that some children have a tendency to bully others who stand out as different in some way – and having epilepsy is certainly one of those ways. The staff at my own old school would certainly have known about my condition, on grounds of safety alone, but they made nothing of it. Would it have

31

been better, it seems strange to wonder, if I had
been bullied, at least to some extent? Given
experiences in adult life, I might have been better
prepared for what was to come. Yet I've seen the
abject misery to which bullying, on the most trivial
of points, can drive a young person, and some not so
young. So what's the answer to my dilemma? No
matter how much I think it over, I honestly don't
know.

4: AFTER THE CATASTROPHE

I'm convinced that there's no-one, whatever the circumstances, who doesn't feel in a sense devalued by unemployment. To lose professional status, after all the years I'd worked to gain it, simply added an extra layer to this sense. When the cause of this action taken against me was no more than a trivial medical problem which I couldn't possibly have brought on myself (although this was almost how I'd been treated), a feeling of unreality set in. Nonetheless, this was how it was.

I discovered most of the facts about lingering social attitudes to epilepsy only well after my letter of disbarment. Most important, however, was to gain any coping mechanisms that I could. What mattered most at the time was, of course: newly married, how was I to support two people, stripped without warning of my income? It's possibly old-fashioned, but a married man still usually feels especially lessened by a loss of ability to look after his family. However, I knew some of this territory well already. In many ways, it's like discovering the bare truth of popular views of epilepsy. Put simply, you either confront them or you lie down and let them crush you. I knew what my choice had to be: I wouldn't let them crush me, but my real regrets I felt for those who suffered because of attitudes to my condition. Like me, they had done nothing to bring this on their heads - very much the opposite.

We found some way or another to manage, usually relying on the most basic unemployment allowances. We forgot the taste of coffee and even, at times, made do with cold water for almost all purposes, personal washing included. Quite simply, we had no choice in the matter.

At last, a year later, an opportunity arose. My disbarment didn't apply to higher education, only schools. Did a local college perhaps have a vacancy for me? Almost incredibly, there was one, teaching my specialist subjects. I was told when appointed that the vacancy was, strictly speaking, only temporary. However, that was no more than a technicality. I could count on my post becoming permanent at the end of the year.

Delighted, I got to work immediately, lecturing to classes of students between eighteen and sixty-five or older, often now retired shipyard workers who wanted to make up for a bad or shortened childhood education, a realisation in them that I especially admired.

They - and the college - deserved my loyalty. I threw into my work everything I had, as the autumn and the year's end drew on.

Then, in early December, came a formal letter: I was to be re-interviewed for the post. Re-interview? Probably - surely - that was no more than a part of the technicalities on the way to being made permanent. Yet, something inside me made me feel uneasy. Hardly surprising, I decided, after the shock of formal disbarment the year earlier. I put any worries to one side as far as I possibly could.

The day came at last. On a dull, grey afternoon, the misty panorama of the city just visible from the third-storey windows, I found myself in a waiting room with five or six others, obviously competitors. I did my best, all I could, to quell a sick fear. Surely they must be applying for different posts? Yes, that must be the answer. It had to be. Hadn't a promise been made? Those words, these thoughts, beat endlessly within my mind, like the sound of a drum in the distance.

I found myself eventually in a room facing a board of elderly men. Questions were asked and notes taken. Some quiet muttering went on and I was then informed of their decision. By all means, the work I'd done was outstanding. However, they couldn't be sure I'd reach pension age. These were almost meaningless words for a man at the time not yet thirty. Even as early as this in my life, were they simply disposing of me almost as a waste product? Yet they admitted themselves that I'd given good service, not to mention past achievements. My position was straightforward enough for their purposes. The many thousands of millions of perfectly serviceable cells making up my brain counted for nothing when set against a few which occasionally misfired.

Their voices droned on: for the reason given, I couldn't be considered for the permanent position. In other words, a promise had been thrown away and forgotten since, in effect, I wasn't a good insurance risk - or so they claimed. And against this broken undertaking I hadn't so much as a trace of redress.

My head of department, I discovered later, who was himself disabled following an accident, had made a special plea on my behalf, but with no effect. At the end of December, I was to leave, whatever might have been guaranteed only a few months earlier.

The journey home that evening is one of my most ghastly memories. The Christmas decorations flickering everywhere seemed to be mocking me at the thought of the poisoned gift waiting for me at the Christmas break. But there was worse to come. How would I tell my wife that our hopes had collapsed again? I did find myself actually considering not even returning home. But I knew there was no choice, however bitter the prospect.

Even by then, I was developing the hardened shell which continues to ensure that it's very difficult to use my disability to offend me. But when others, close to me, are affected, it's a very different matter.

Eventually my feet, moving artificially slowly, brought me to our door. Inside, I could hear my wife contentedly singing to herself. I would have done anything just to turn around and move away. But I knew that was what I couldn't, and mustn't do.

When I did give my news, the reaction was as dreadful as I could have feared. There were at first torrents of tears, then that particular silence, worse even than the tears, that comes of utter wretchedness.

It was partly to escape from this hideous atmosphere at home that I did return to work the next day. Now, however, I put only minimal effort into it. What I could avoid doing, I didn't do. A promise made to me had been broken and cast aside. Why should I keep my side of the bargain? At least for the time being, I was being paid more than a pittance to keep us alive. But Christmas was drawing on, and day by day the thought of what hung over us grew. How would we manage now? What would the new year bring?

The answer to that question was straightforward enough. The new year meant the beginning of four years of unemployment. Application after application failed, running eventually into hundreds, almost always on the ground of my state of health, or, more commonly, what others thought it was. I could find almost no-one who would accept the reality: that the epilepsy was rarely more than a passing nuisance. I practically never collapsed or lost my balance because of it. It was no more just a short flickering of awareness from time to time.

After some time, I was outraged to find even a disability employment officer actually blaming me, in effect, for what had happened, whatever effort I had put into my past work. I'd had two bites of the cherry, hadn't I? He asked, leaning back in his chair with an attitude which struck me at least as close to contempt. Yes, I replied, but sour cherries they'd turned out to be, not worth the effort which I'd undeniably put into picking them. Could he argue with that point? As I'd expected, he struggled to find a reply - and that's how I left him as I stood and walked out of his office, saying nothing further.

I never spoke to this man again or replied to invitations to further interviews with him. He had shown contempt and insult, and that showed the true nature of the man. And so I had nothing to say to him. Any belief I might earlier have had - and I had - in him had evaporated. I too had my pride, as does anyone else, disabled or not. And that in itself deserved respect, from him or anyone else. Any person may have some particular characteristic, say disability of whatever kind, but this is only part of the entire person. There's much more besides - if someone cares to look for it. The disability officer had committed a cardinal error, which I couldn't forgive. He'd treated a part of me as more important than the whole. He was someone in a position to know better. So why should I speak to him again, if I couldn't be sure he wasn't doing the same, even covertly, on another occasion? What he had said that day was quite enough to condemn him, as far as I was concerned.

I've never had a place in my life for bitterness. I think of it as the most negative and destructive of emotions. No-one emerges the better from expressing, even simply feeling, it - least of all, I believe, the embittered person. Since that interview, many years ago, I've asked myself repeatedly whether that was an occasion when I failed to keep my standard. But no, I had to make my point: that I resented what had been said or implied to me, and was fully prepared to hit back.

Disabled I might be, but that didn't mean meek and powerless too.

For whatever reason, there are some medical conditions that are sometimes seen as the personal failing of the person with them, regardless of the difficulties they may cause him. One of these conditions, I've often observed, is epilepsy. Perhaps this is partly because it at least resembles drunkenness. And perhaps there's something far more basic in human nature in how the matter has long been viewed, as I can illustrate shortly.

In refusing to have another meeting with the disability officer, I believe I'd done something to make my point: that I wasn't prepared timidly just to accept this attitude, and especially not from someone who surely had been trained to understand my plight better. I treated him as he treated me. He deserved no better. To write these words saddens me, even now. But to this day, I won't accept denigration on the ground of my medical condition. My determination has only strengthened with time. To have a medical difficulty makes me no-one's inferior, only slightly different. It's nothing more than that. And that rule applies to disability in general: to be disabled is to have a difference from what's normally considered usual. It has nothing - and should have nothing - to do with anyone's sense of self-esteem or abilities. A disabled person has the burden of coping in an able-bodied world. That, I've learned, is no mean task - and something to take a pride in when achieved. To make this point isn't to be aggressive or embittered. Instead, the disabled person must learn one vital skill above all: self-confidence. And, at appropriate times, he must be prepared to assert himself.

5: WORK NOT IN PROGRESS

It almost certainly must seem a paradox to any reader. It is true, however, to say that this interview actually did much to save me from total despair. Whatever presumptions might have been wrongly made by others, the grim prophecy now made of my premature death was something I simply couldn't take seriously. It's perhaps instructive, and I find myself shaking my head from to time over the fact, that I have just passed the standard retirement age, which that elderly group of interviewers assured me I would never live to see (on what possible evidence I was never to find out). Nothing, I've come to believe, is written in stone before you see it actually carved before your eyes. And that includes the notion that people with epilepsy are fated to an early death. It can happen, as it can with others, but isn't common. Scepticism can often pay dividends. Had I really heard said what I had? If so, I wasn't prepared to accept it.

For some time, therefore, I found myself protected from depression by my utter bemusement, a sense of unreality. Not, however, entirely. There still is a tendency among some of the population, those not in that position themselves, to refer to the unemployed as 'idle'. In fact, for a high proportion, a period of unemployment is frantic with activity. There's, of course, the struggle to find other work.

41

But more than that: there's the question of finding ways to fill the empty hours. This is something we rarely hear mentioned, but there's no denying it's a very real problem. Not every minute of the day can possibly be spent in thinking of hitting on just the right opportunity for work. There has to be a diversion of some sort. But what? Even if there is one, can it be afforded? This is a difficulty familiar too for many once busy, but now retired, people. What are they to do with their days now? For both groups, the world has suddenly changed, and not necessarily to their liking.

And this, following the broken promise of a permanent position, was the situation I now found myself in, yet again. It should all have been so different, if others had kept their word. However, they hadn't, and, except in my own mind, I was fit only for the spoil-heap, with not the slightest hope of redress. So, what now? I just didn't know.

It was particularly difficult with two people concerned, living on a pathetic unemployment allowance. My family helped, by all means, but we lived at a considerable distance from them, and only my father, then still working, could drive. This meant that help could come only at the weekends, or sometimes in the evening.

I don't think it's too fanciful or extravagant to compare life in unemployment with being sentenced to wear an electronic tag for an offence committed. Lack of any but the most basic income, far smaller and less generous than the general public is sometimes led to believe, puts very real limits on what can be done or where anyone can go, as if just another form of surveillance, but with a very real and important difference. Someone sentenced to wear a surveillance tag at least knows the time he must serve before it's removed. This is something the unemployed person can't begin even to guess at: how long is this state of things going to last? And even, as time passes, the fear grows: will this ever end? Will it always be like this? Will he ever have a normal life? It's impossible to avoid these fears, most of all in the evenings and at night, when there's nothing to distract attention from the situation. It's vital to find an interest which will take your mind from the subject. Over the cause of the problem, a slight medical difficulty, the person with that difficulty has no influence whatever. Among his few ways of helping himself is not allowing himself to dwell on the matter.

There's another comparison too between the life of anyone wearing a tag and someone's who's unemployed. The general public, or a considerable number, commonly feel that they have a right to pass moral judgements on both groups, with nothing like a full knowledge of the facts of the matter. Where the unemployed are concerned, the usual call is that they should get up and find work. But that's exactly what so many are trying to do, again and again.

It's especially galling to hear such comments from critics you've far outperformed and who have no knowledge – or sometimes even interest – in quite why you're not earning a living in the conventional way.

Covert disabilities, such as epilepsy, are especially prone to such condemnation. There's no choice, however, but to learn to bear it. And how do you find a way round the problem of disclosing the very health condition which cost you your work in the first place? Refer to it, experience teaches you very quickly, and you can practically count on rejection. However, if you don't refer to it, when the health condition is eventually discovered, you face the threat of dismissal as untrustworthy or unreliable. That, naturally, means even less opportunity of finding another opening. You're caught, in other words, between the two jaws of invisible pincers - invisible, but only too real.

This was probably the most unhelpful medical advice I ever received, at a regular meeting with a consultant. I explained to him in outline the difficulties of finding work for someone with epilepsy. Yes, he agreed, my situation was 'unenviable' - a gross understatement, I thought, but didn't say so. I suspect, however, my expression left no doubt of what was in my mind. What I could do, he brightly suggested, was just not disclose my health condition in an application.

I couldn't believe what I was hearing from someone of his background. In work, it would be only a matter of time until the condition showed itself. It would be even less time under the strain of trying to conceal the signs of the epilepsy which I didn't disclose. Eventually, someone would notice something strange in my behaviour, perhaps even something I wasn't aware of myself. It was this meeting that led me to keep detailed notes of my seizures, so as to give as clear a picture as I could of the reality of the matter, and to make sure that medical advisers were given a copy at future meetings. This is something which I still do.

There's a mismatch between the lives lived by medical specialists and the lives lived by the people who have the condition, day by day, on which the specialists give advice. This has to be bridged somehow, and this is what I try to do by providing notes and reports with as much detail as possible. Textbooks as used by specialists certainly have their place. However, the hard personal experiences, not just the medical aspects, but the social problems which the condition can give rise to, aren't likely to be mentioned in texts about brain functions. Epilepsy, too, is so unpredictable and wayward that it's impossible to present it for inspection. We don't know when it's going to strike, and in what way. Leave even an outline description of it for more than an hour or two, and it can easily be almost impossible to detail. Like a dream, it has no meaning outside itself, and so is quickly forgotten.

This is probably the best solution: to keep almost immediate notes of what the specialist isn't likely to see, still less feel. That's no fault of his, if he doesn't have the condition himself (which is highly unlikely). Barring artificially stimulated seizures, which have been performed on volunteers in Canada, for example, second-hand information, as detailed as possible, is the only way. At least one neurologist who bravely agreed to have an artificial attack in the temporal lobe under supervision emerged shocked from the experience. It was something of such a nature, she admitted to her credit, that she could never have imagined.

The health of both of us was gradually deteriorating and, even more troubling, home life became brittle. We submerged ourselves in the world of books and read for hours a day. Even this, however, carried risks. Discussion of the most trivial aspects of some work could easily flare up in major disagreements. Too long together in any one day, as we were now forced to be, meant we were grating against one another, reflecting on the negative aspects of each other's character, never the positive which had brought us together.

Strangely, something which never caused any real disputes was my love of early mythology, which my wife came to share early on. It's tragic that this is a subject that's so often dismissed as nothing but a collection of children's stories and has practically vanished from the school curriculum. While teaching, I had always made a point of referring to it.

In fact, the enormous range of mythology represents basic truths in a pictorial manner, rather like a biblical parable. There's a deep sense of encouragement and comfort in finding in stories thousands of years old difficulties so like those which you're undergoing yourself in the present day. This tells you that you're not alone, that others have been through the same experiences, if possibly in a different way. If they were literally true or not didn't matter in the slightest. At least the problems were mentioned, and hints given at possible solutions. If the matter could be mentioned, even symbolically, then clearly someone else had been there before, possibly only in thought or perhaps in reality. With myth, that's not what's important. It's the myth which matters and the ideas which develop from it.

I still keep up my love of myth and have found it greatly valuable in troubling times. I'm not at all surprised that at least one branch of psychology relies heavily on myth. We can speak about abstracts, say loyalty or endurance, but how does our mind picture them? The answer's simple: it can't. What it can do, however, is imagine actions or figures (Jung's 'archetypes') which are loyal or enduring. It's these which come to us in dreams. My research thesis had dealt with the psychological effect of early myth. Without exaggeration, it's easily possible that it's to this I owe my mental stability at that hideous time. Add to that my love of ancient history, something else to absorb myself in.

More and more as time passes, I become convinced that the contemptuous dismissal of myth from education over recent years in favour of something more supposedly 'relevant' has a great deal to do with the rootlessness of so many young people. Many other societies, including some which we dismiss as 'primitive', prize their mythologies. Mythological concepts lie at the very base of human thought, one of the main reasons that so many mythologies in so many different areas often have much in common. Cut people, the younger people in particular, adrift from those basics and the only result can be rootlessness. It stands to reason that a plant can't grow if it's cut away from its root. The present is meaningless - rootless - unless it's based on its past.

I frequently used mythology in my teaching days. It rarely failed to fix pupils' attention, no matter what their own ethnic or other background was. A particular pride of mine was when a school pupil, only just short of being illiterate, asked to borrow a reference book on the subject, not easy reading by any means. Quite literally within weeks, his parents told me, he was transfixed and soon had reached at least the standard level for his age. He'd found just the right stimulation. After some time, the reference book he'd borrowed was returned to me, with a strange white ring on the green cover. His parents apologised for this, but there was no need. For both the borrower and me, it spelled success. It was where he'd put his cocoa mug each night before drifting off to sleep, bringing the book with him to bed. I've been careful to keep this book, for in a sense it proves what I had to say about mythology. We can always struggle on, aiming to succeed. I can't think of a more relevant message in the complex, troubled world of today.

That both of us were too much in one another's company, however, resulted in my inventing false interviews. I hoarded small change from the shopping to cover transport costs to the nearest city and, if possible, enough to buy a cup of coffee. This would allow me a few hours on my own. I was used to long walks and, in a city, there were so many distractions, even possible suggestions for breaking out of our situation. I don't know what my wife did at these times. I don't think, however, that I

48

was greatly selfish or dishonest in doing what I did. She too needed time to herself, time to think her own thoughts. Did she guess at the truth of what I was doing? I'm sure she must have. It must have struck her as strange that none of these supposed interviews was followed by a letter of acceptance or rejection. Yet nothing was ever said about this. Most probably, she longed for her hours on her own as much as I did for myself.

Several times, on the journey home, I found myself shaken awake by the bus driver, well past my intended stop. Three times, our local doctor diagnosed nervous exhaustion. At home, I was noticed slowly sliding from a chair to the floor. It wasn't epilepsy, but weariness. The question was now glaringly straightforward: how much longer could this last? How much more could either of us take? When would the breaking point come?

There's an important point that must be made. Why didn't my family help more than they did? I must stress that they're not at all to blame. It was my own senseless pride that prevented me from telling them the truth of the matter. If a man couldn't look after his family, I told myself, he shouldn't have a family. My then wife's health was failing too. She was unable to work now and contribute to the family income. The problem of providing was up to me, and me alone. Doing that was my duty, and I was failing to carry it out.

There's very little that can be done for exhaustion. Its effects could easily be passed off as the consequences of epileptic attacks. This wasn't entirely untruthful. Both of us were becoming debilitated. Debility meant more seizures, and seizures were, and are now, exhausting. It was a ghastly and apparently unbreakable cycle of cause and effect.

It was only many years later - and even then I felt embarrassed - that I told my family, who had formed the growing impression at that time that more was untoward than I was prepared to admit, the full truth. They were shocked, including at my past unwillingness to tell them the facts of the matter. The responsibility for this failure had been entirely mine.

Yet, there's perhaps some reality in the truism, that even in the darkness of nights there's a glimmer of light. We only have to wait, difficult though it may be. In our case, this took the form of a mysterious letter arriving one early December morning. Would we, it asked, be attending the ceremony? There was that and little else.

Ceremony? What ceremony? At that time of the year, this had surely to be some form of advertisement. With this in mind, we went over the letter line by line. Yet it mentioned nothing for sale, still less cost. Eventually, bewildered, we simply left it lying on the kitchen table. It had been addressed to me, so there was plainly no postal error. What, then, was it? We simply couldn't prevent ourselves individually picking it up and reading it over again, and again, but each time with the same result.

The mystery was unravelled at last only a few days later. I received word that my research thesis had been accepted after the regular prolonged examination. The letters had simply arrived in reverse order. We could barely stop laughing. And there was an emotion too which went much deeper than laughter. We had only to check the familiar telephone number on the first letter – and it hadn't occurred to us to do even that.

I don't think it's really possible for me to explain to anyone else the full effect of the arrival of such a letter. The glow which filled me then, when I had read the award letter several times, has never left me, even after many years. More, however, than that: it brought tumbling back memory after memory of my years, which I had loved, as a research student. I had begun, under persistent difficulties, actually to doubt their very existence, but now I had all the evidence of their reality which I needed.

But there was more, which added layers to such a treasure. The first was the awareness that the bulk of my thesis, two-thirds or so, I had persisted in writing to take my mind from the sheer bleakness of our circumstances and prospects. Secondly – for which I still thank the awarding authorities – there was a paragraph in the letter accompanying the degree. They had been aware, they said, of special difficulties in my life. Nonetheless, they had felt no reason on that ground to make me any special allowances. I must be treated just as anyone else. This is what I still want, not to be patronised by special pleading.

With those words, my dismissal as in effect a non-person just a few years earlier crumbled away (not that I had ever accepted it, in any case). Could anyone now argue that I hadn't proved myself the

51

equal and more, on the same territory, as my detractors, and so proved them in the wrong? At that particular time, my extra degree might not yet have practical value. Psychologically, however, its effect, on both my family and me, was immense and remained so. It hangs even now on my wall, as a symbol of the meaninglessness of the term disability. This, it seems to tell me, is what I did in the grimmest of circumstances – and could do again. What concerns me is what I can, not what I can't, do – and this viewpoint I recommend to disabled people as a whole. We all, disabled or not, have within us a reservoir of endurance and ability which often go unnoticed. It's for us to discover it – and to ignore apparent obstacles, including not least the human variety.

Family celebrations followed, of course. This was only a first step on the way back to a normal life, but it was, I continue to believe, a major and deeply meaningful one, regardless of what might or what not might follow.

6: RELEASE

I still clearly remember that Saturday mid-evening, almost four years after the breaking of the college's promise, that the phone rang at our home. It was a school friend in past years, well familiar with my position. He'd noticed, he said, while waiting on a railway platform, an advert placed in a newspaper by a school in the north of England, looking for a specialist in my field. I might just be interested in following this up.

One advantage of a hopeless situation is that the person in it is insulated against disappointment. But school work? It occurred to me then that my disbarment didn't apply in England. But would that make the slightest difference? Surely not, with an employment history like mine.

There was as little to lose as there was to gain, I thought, as I wrote a letter of application. It was all the more startling, therefore, to receive a week or two later an invitation to interview. The fare would be expensive, but only just manageable, and I agreed to attend.

The interview seemed to go well, even though I made no secret of my past and my health condition. The questions asked were relevant and to the point. I answered in the same way and returned home that same evening.

I only occasionally received refusals in writing, so was mildly surprised when a letter arrived for me, postmarked where I had been interviewed. But this was different. It wasn't a refusal, but an invitation to re-interview.

Re-interview? Hadn't I heard that word before, when my untimely death was predicted? But this time the context was different. I wasn't already on the staff of the place where re-interview was requested. What did this mean?

I felt a surge of nausea, which I later came to recognise for what it was. It was the rebirth of hope, however slight. Nothing would come of it, I knew well, for nothing ever did. However, there it was. If it was no more than a shadow of opportunity, I had to grasp at it.

I attended the re-interview some weeks later. It went much as before, but with one major difference. The impossible had happened. Against all the odds, I'd been appointed as from early autumn. I was evidently best qualified for the vacancy. Could this be true, I asked myself time after time on the long way home. But if I had doubts – and I had many, perhaps understandably – the appointment letter was in my grasp.

Commuting such a distance was out of the question. We cancelled the tenancy of the place where we'd lived for that appalling four years and moved south to within a mile or two of where I'd be working from now on. The memory of the original flat disappearing into the distance as we moved away carries no kindly sentiments for me. It was more as if I'd finally found the opportunity to wash my hands of the entire district. It was finished and behind us at last.

Finding a place to rent in the city to which we'd moved was almost unbelievably simple. It was, I remember, a cottage dating back to the Victorian era, with two storeys and with gardens all around. From the upper storey, we could actually see part of the school where I'd be working from now on. It would be a healthy walk in the mornings and evenings and at weekends into the city itself.

My first term there began. Any place which would accept me deserved my loyalty. Evening after evening, I brought back work for correction. However, this was something which I enjoyed doing. My wife's health hadn't quite been restored, so that I did have to help her out. The improvements in her state, nonetheless, were obvious and growing. There was nothing now for me to blame myself for, as I had been doing for some years.

It's a strange thing, completely beyond all reason. Commonly, a man who's deprived of work and some means of supporting his family, even if he has no responsibility for the loss (for example, when I found myself the victim of a broken promise), will tend, little by little, to turn the sense of guilt inwards. It may be perfectly obvious that you've done, and are still doing, everything possible, but if you're not managing when others are, then somehow the fault lies with you. It's something like the attitude of Boxer the carthorse in George Orwell's *Animal Farm*. Whenever some crisis arises, his response is the same: that he must get up a little earlier from now on and work harder each day. That fine intent doesn't, however, save him from his final journey to the knacker's yard. If anything, it brings it nearer.

Is this every male's attitude in this situation, and only the male's, not the female's too? I don't know, for I've never asked. It does seem likely, however, that it's a view shared by at least some of both sexes, for not only men have a conscience or a sense of failure.

For me, however, none of that mattered any more. I could make up for lost time now. In the first few months, I helped pupils secure around fifteen scholarships. At parents' meetings, I was thanked for rekindling their children's interests in my subjects. Might it even be possible, I was asked, to expand them and bring in other, associated subjects? I'd certainly look into it, I replied, but those decisions didn't lie with me. I'd have to ask the school headmaster.

One Monday morning, just before the Easter break, he asked me for some advice on the following year's curriculum. I'd managed at last to secure some status. The matters parents had asked me about were put to him. He'd consider it, he said, but within the limits of the school's finances. At home, we began to speak of a possible holiday, a laughable notion only the year before. Perhaps this destination, or perhaps that? If anyone needed a holiday, we did. And now one was at last in prospect.

Mid-week, a note came to me one morning from the headmaster. He'd like to speak to me in his office during the afternoon break. His deputy would be present too. Probably, I told myself, he'd reached his decision on what I'd asked.

Or had he? Slowly, as the hours passed, I fought back another possibility. It was absurd, I knew. Hadn't I been consulted as his specialist only two days before? Obviously, surely, all he wanted was more detail on the future curriculum. The day passed with agonising slowness. I revised over and over the information I had provided on Monday.

Then it was afternoon break, as I realised with a shock. Already late, I made my way down to his office, deliberately slowly, yet desperate to shake off another thought. He invited me to enter his office and sit down. Somehow I knew what was coming, but could never have guessed the whole story. It was with deep regret, I heard him say as if from some far distance, that he'd have to dismiss me. It was at least possible that I could be viewed as a threat to safety, in particular in case of fire.

Fire? But I dealt with words and books. I may have tried to make some reply, but from the icy water in which I seemed to be standing it didn't seem possible. In recognition of my services, he continued, the regular month's notice would be extended to three - until July.

But for the shock I was in, then and later, I would have questioned his logic. If I truly was a threat to safety, I should have been dismissed instantly. Keeping me on for three months, while claiming I endangered safety, was a total contradiction. This was an argument which didn't occur to me, however, until long afterwards. It was a regrettable decision, he said, but he had taken legal advice. In recent years, just for my own curiosity, I've asked a solicitor about the matter. What had been done, he informed me, hadn't been legally justified, even at the time. The claim that a disabled person in some obscure way constitutes a fire hazard remains even now a common pretext for his removal.

The worst was kept for last. I would be spared, he said, the difficulty of bringing the news to my wife. He himself had brought my dismissal letter to her at our home that same morning - before I had any notion that any problem existed. I've since been told that this is a method often employed to give notice of a serviceman's death in action.

Brought the word to her first, hours earlier, when her health was only slowly returning? I was so plainly shocked that it was evident I couldn't continue that day. His deputy drove me home, the last thing on Earth I wanted. Anywhere but home. But what was the choice?

I knew in hideous detail what I dreaded finding on my arrival. But I'd underestimated it vastly. A sunny afternoon, spring flowers only just beginning to bloom. But beyond, on the front doorstep, a crushed personality, crushed now, I somehow knew, beyond all hope. I was left standing helplessly on the pavement, my colleague's muttered words, 'I'm sorry', in my ears, with as little meaning as the whispering of the breeze. There seemed to be a bell tolling in my head, over and over, drowning out the truth at one stroke, emphasising it with the next.

Home life that evening and the next day was, I'm sure, difficult. The truth is, I just don't know.

Nature has its kinder aspects, one of them a sort of anaesthetic. I've lost all memory of that time. I probably should have stayed at home to provide what comfort I could. But wasn't I the difficulty? There was one hellish irony to be faced. The next day, when I returned to work as normal for what would be only a short time longer, was, in the old Roman Catholic calendar, the day dedicated to Saint Joseph the Worker.

At the end of the week, my family collected me from the roadside to bring me to their home for rest. My tenancy had somehow been cancelled. In a week that had begun in a blaze of hope, on one single day, I'd lost my career, my home and my marriage.

7: A CHANGE OF COURSE

I've not the slightest memory of the 120 miles drive back to my family's home for a period of desperately needed rest. My ex-wife went back for that time to her mother. My family have told me that, immediately I reached their home, I went into a series of convulsions, leading them no choice but to call out the emergency doctor. I'm told that he expressed outrage at the way I had been treated by my employer. In the circumstances, I should have been granted a period away from the school to try to regain my health. Of his calling-out, too, I know nothing whatever except for what I've been told. As far as I remember, that was some considerable time after the event. I'm sure, however, I must have been informed shortly afterwards. If so, I know nothing whatever about it.

My employer, as far as I'm aware, had never suggested this possibility of a period of rest. I'd been coping, although I had been acting as my wife's carer to some extent after the working day. I saw the dismissal letter brought to my ex-wife at our then home that dreadful day. It listed a number of attacks I'd suffered. None of them, however, could realistically be regarded as serious. As far as I knew, no-one had even mentioned them to me at the time of occurrence. I'd received the *coup de grace*, with a single concession in respect of services performed or as a special consideration of some other circumstance: extended notice, which defied all logic or sense. Or was this simply a device just to win time to search for my replacement? Who knows?

If I hadn't performed satisfactorily, I would normally have been informed in the strongest terms. But nothing of the sort had happened, if anything the opposite. I'm driven to one conclusion, however painful I find it even now: my colleagues had seen me as an embarrassment. This was an attitude which I'd experienced before, and since, and not only in employment. In or out of employment, it's one which must change, for people with epilepsy in general, or for us there's no such thing as security. We hear constantly that we live in a free society. Certain minorities, not least the disabled, have every right to question that opinion. I believe that my experiences as described justify this claim.

Naturally, it wasn't possible or even realistic for me to remain unaffected by our recent experience, the destruction of our entire way of life and the sudden loss of all expectations of only a few weeks, or rather days, before. Day after day, family members, when leaving for work, would place my daily medication on the bedside table. On their return, in the early evening, I was regularly found still fast asleep since the night before, my medication untouched. I had been left stunned, of which a natural consequence was shock.

With time, still at my family's home, I took to idly drawing and painting, mainly mythological scenes. A lost home, a lost marriage, a lost career

61

just didn't seem to matter. Even when a solicitor's letter arrived, warning me to remove my property from what had been our home by a given date or the locks would be changed, like the rest of what had happened it was as if it all belonged on a different world. It had no relevance to anything, and to humane standards least of all. I simply brushed it aside.

My long walks began again after some days. I was in parks familiar from long before, or in museums and art galleries, where the exhibits seemed almost like childhood friends. Luckily it was a warm spring that year. I was walking by a riverside estuary, no great distance from where I'd gone to school many years before. The sunlight was still playing on the waves just as I remembered, more and more as the tides emptied the river waters into the Irish Sea. As they had been when I'd attended school, long-derelict fishing boats lay abandoned on the sand banks, still where I remembered them.

These represented, I thought at first, almost a metaphor for my own experiences. Farther on still were the small peninsulas, densely covered with broad-leaf trees. No, nothing was changed here. These were timeless constants, things I could rely on, just like the hills lying beyond the opposite bank, where once I'd gone exploring years before. It wasn't these, I soon came to realise, which had failed me; it was certain people, social concepts, which had done so.

That flickering of sunlight on the water, day after day, fed slowly through my eyes and into my brain. Something strange, I gradually realised, was taking place. As time passed, my sense of fatalism, then despair, was crystallising into its precise opposite: determination. Perhaps it's not a coincidence that both sides of the same coin, both the negative and the positive terms, begin with the same syllable. If even the tides could be constant, couldn't I be too? Why not? As the time passed, this sense only grew stronger. Determination hardened further, into a sense of defiance. How else to confront these people, these concepts? There was no other way.

The month-long Easter break saw me, after all, packing to return. Only weeks earlier, I just hadn't cared about going back to that northern town. What would be the point, I thought then, if it would be no more, in practice, than to attend my own funeral rites? No, I gradually reasoned, there was more at stake. The best time to strike back at an opponent (for this was how I now viewed my employer) was surely when he thought me crushed, beyond all hope. I had no choice in honour but to prove him wrong.

I didn't deceive myself that there was the slightest chance of reinstatement. However, there was another vital aspect to the matter, one second to none: it was my own self-respect. I could be sure that I would go down in time, but I would stand my ground, disability or no disability. My employer would have no argument against that, for I wasn't prepared to allow him one. Let him make of that whatever he would. He must surely be taught a lesson.

Our one-time home was, of course, now lost. However, I wanted nothing less than to see it again. The memories and associations it would convey would be too raw and painful, as is still the case decades later. Somehow I secured my property again. I worked out my notice from a cheap boarding house with a minimum of facilities, walking, as before, the two or three miles there and back. I wasn't going to give way.

Parents met me a number of times and let me know that they'd made known their sense of indignation to the school headmaster at his impending disposal of me. If they were prepared to accept me, why wasn't he? It was just the epilepsy enigma yet again, in another of its endless variations.

Their words were gratifying, and I respect their sentiments, even now, so many years after the event. Protest, however, as they might, what they were doing amounted to demanding a reprieve, but only after the prisoner had already been executed. It was no more than a gesture, but one which I greatly appreciate.

No place on Earth is worse for keeping secrets than a school, any school. By one means or another, the pupils had found out too that my stay would be limited. In their own way, one just as meaningful as their parents' way, they made their annoyance known. Who would take my place? I couldn't answer that question. Possibly no-one could as yet.

My colleagues' attitude was rather different. If I entered the staff room, they commonly looked away and clearly pretended to become engaged in deep conversations, one with another. I didn't sense hostility, however. It was more like the behaviour we commonly see when someone realises that he's approaching a recently bereaved neighbour. What's he to say that won't sound false and hollow, or perhaps even sanctimonious? Better to say nothing at all, yet that seems uncivil. Or was there perhaps, in some at least, a thoroughly deserved sense of guilt? If there was, let them live with it, for I was the last person prepared to offer them comfort.

Even for some years later, when I unwittingly came down the same streets as an ex-colleague, I noticed that almost without exception, he would suddenly notice something intensely interesting in a nearby shop window, however unlikely that might be where some shops were concerned. I simply would go on my way and notice from the corner of my eye his head turning when I appeared to be at a reasonably safe distance. It can be remarkably instructive in social terms to be one of the living dead, as I now appeared to be

For the rest of my period of notice, I spent little time in the staff room and went walking around out of doors. Luckily, it was a picturesque building and a historical city and the warm spell continued. Within easy walking distance, there was a calm river, budding trees lining its banks.

Not that the warm spring was necessarily a blessing. The lengthening days and growing sunlight formed an unwelcome contrast to my own shortening tenure and the bleakness of my future, whatever that might be. It's obviously painful to find yourself in a place where you've loved to work, knowing how soon you have no choice but to leave. A distraction was needed. Yet again, that became walking and reading.

It was my last day, the day just before the summer break, that proved truly hideous. I arrived as usual, determined to face it out. Throughout the entire day, it was as if I was observing events from behind a sheet of plate glass. Somehow I was separated from what was going on, while yet directly facing it. I seemed to hear with complete clarity conversations taking place a hundred metres or so away. Words spoken nearby appeared to have taken on a ringing, vibrating quality.

Only later, I found that a particular colleague had been deputed that day specifically to take care of me. I now recognise that, under the strain, I must have been experiencing seizure after seizure, probably relatively mild. The apparent ringing quality in nearby sound at such times is especially familiar as an indicator of seizures, especially at the beginning of onset.

Even in that state, I was aware of a strange contradiction. Why would they show such care now, when a little more concern earlier on in my time there could have made such a difference? It was all so utterly senseless and contradictory. It was my seizures which were the claimed ground for my dismissal, yet the awareness of my dismissal had brought on the seizures that day. Where was the sense in all this? The answer to that question was blunt and to the point. There was no sense in the matter. If it was genuinely believed that I represented a fire risk, as had been claimed only a few months before, bringing about personal disaster, shouldn't I have been requested not to attend the closing day of term?

At last, mercifully, it was all at an end and the place fell quiet. I made my way to the staff room to pick up my remaining belongings. One colleague muttered to me, 'Such a wretched illness', and some other words which I couldn't follow. I ignored him and his remarks, something which I now regret doing. This was an attempt at a gesture of kindness, I now realise. I should have treated him better in return, whatever the circumstances. And yet, hadn't I made my point? Strained or not, now possibly to a medically inadvisable level, I hadn't permitted myself not to attend what I knew would be sure to prove an immensely trying day. This determination, or call it defiance, is still, for me, a matter of pride. I could have pleaded illness, but had refused to do so.

It was what was waiting for me when I went down to my classroom which had the greatest effect. Together with a short note to wish me well for the future, there was a gift waiting for me, to which all my registration pupils, of a mean age of about twelve, had contributed. In one way they had been observant, less so in another. It was a delicately painted ashtray, together with a sympathetic note. Yes, I was and remain enthusiastic about the arts, but I've never smoked in my life. Somehow, that seemed to compensate for the rest of the day while, surely unintentionally, providing an ironic counterpoint to the grounds for my dismissal in the first place. The gift of an ashtray to a non-smoking supposed fire risk! It was impossible not to smile.

I've kept the ashtray, still unused, carefully put away for safety. After walking back that evening to my rented room, I had to realise that, for whatever reason, my passion for providing education wasn't mutual as far as potential employers were concerned. What now? I had no choice: I was going to have to speak again to a disablement rehabilitation officer, whatever the outcome.

8: BACK TO THE DRAWING BOARD

Had my experiences to then left me without bitterness? To claim that they hadn't done so, up to a point, would surely mark me out as something less than human, not more. A career, a marriage, a home destroyed in a matter of hours, without warning or sensible cause: what else could I feel but resentment, anger and, deeper down, a desire for revenge?

I don't think, even so many years later, that those emotions have quite left me. It would be a pious pretence for me to claim otherwise after what I had seen done to my then family. Why shouldn't I wish for redress? It was surely only normal. Yet I could expect no redress, for there was none. Why had we been subjected to others' disastrous and outright stupidity without good cause? If I had shown signs of tiredness, as I very probably had, as a result of leaving work in the evenings to become, at least to a point, my then wife's carer, why had no questions been asked, no offer made of leave of absence? It's possibly suggestive that, while I myself had taken barely any time from work, if any, one of my successors had, I was told by an ex-colleague, needed several months' sick leave not long after taking over my post. There could be only one conclusion: some conditions were, or still are, more acceptable than others.

My gesture of defiance in returning to complete my term of extended notice had, of course, contained at least an element of resentment. Think what my employer might, or perhaps did, I was more than ready to meet him as at least his equal. He would learn to his cost, I determined, what he was simply casting aside. Yet there was another consideration: embitterment is always destructive and corrosive, to the embittered person above all. Even in childhood, I had seen it many times in various places, still with no idea of quite what I was then observing. And Goodwill Square, years later, had forced the message home. Those shouts of fury, the screams of terror in the semi-darkness, the pointlessly sacrificed young life; the memory had never left me. It remains with me even now. I've tried twice to exorcise the memory by revisiting the place, now peaceful for many years, but the very sight of the signpost at the entry filled me, quite literally, with nausea, forcing me to turn away each time. It had become that evening a symbol of bitterness and hatred, sickening even though understandable at the time. The very thought of revisiting our old street provokes similar emotions, so that I've never returned there. The memories remain as vivid as they ever were.

Yet I've now realised that experience in the past had in its own strange way actually helped me in my later life. On the afternoon that I had been deposited by my colleague at our garden gate and forced to witness what I had, it was not the first time that I had seen what was by any standard unacceptable, even inhuman. No-one can be truly hardened to such experiences, but we can be prepared – to some extent – for them to happen.

After my final day, then, I was left with a simple choice: to brood on the wrong done to us, or to occupy myself in some other way. My usual choice, of walking for hours in what is a picturesque city, was of great help, but only for so long each day. When evening, then darkness, came, what was I to do then? I might brood, harmfully perhaps most of all to me, on the harm done, or do what I did: read incessantly. Book after book after book – the titles scarcely mattered. I revisited my old textbooks, all of which I had kept from years before.

Yet there was a very practical consideration: as my savings ran out, how was I to live? I eventually forced myself to do what I had long known I had no choice but to do: revisit a disability resettlement officer. From past experience, this was scarcely something to anticipate with anything like relish.

At least the officer himself was a considerable improvement on his predecessor, whom I had boycotted rather than accept further insult. He was friendly, good company and in good spirits, practically jovial. Yet practical solutions to my predicament, even he had to admit, were anything but simple to come by. Would I, he asked, be prepared to accept menial work? That depended, I replied, on quite what he meant by 'menial'. Perhaps work in an office – if he could find any available, for, he had to admit, my condition put limits on the types of work for which I might be suited. At least by then I had taught myself the

71

typewriter keyboard, which I could use quickly and accurately, and by now have adapted to word-processing use.

Learning the keyboard had had more than one purpose. The obvious one was to increase my prospects of finding work. The other has gone unmentioned until now. When, finally, I had to admit to myself that my savings could last only a short time longer in the dingy boardings I had occupied since the collapse of my career and all that went with it, I had no choice but to apply for emergency housing, and was lucky enough to find it. This had only an open fire for heating, for someone with epilepsy unusable with any safety. As a precaution, I bought a paraffin heater which was at least advertised as having a foolproof safety attachment. Luckily, the occasion never arose when this safeguard might prove necessary. As winter approached, I found one way of keeping my fingers comparatively warm was to keep them moving on a portable typewriter. Over that first winter, by this method, I produced a three hundred page translation of a work on early history. I had hit on a valuable lesson: I was linking up a skill I already had with a way of coping with a need, to stay warm and, I hoped, to make myself more attractive to a potential employer.

That apart, working on this at least partly kept my attention from the sense of isolation. Not so very long before, I preferred not to remember, it had all been very different. From that, work on translation, not an easy skill, diverted my attention. Whether or not it had any other real purpose simply didn't matter. Even as the days, and my hands, grew warmer, at least I was occupied, working with a skill which I knew I had to maintain and keep fresh. I honestly don't know why, but before and since that time, language had been my passion. Now it was serving me well in return, simply keeping me busy. There was no more to it than that.

I should, I now realise, have asked my family for help, which they would willingly have provided. However, my pride – the same pride which had made me strike back at my ex-employers by defiantly proving them wrong - couldn't accept the thought of making that request. I can speak, obviously, only for a man: once he has left the family home, he knows he must make his own way. Except in extreme need, there's no looking back. He's made his choice and must stand by it. I've sometimes wondered if this is nothing more than personal pride or something more basic, something I find it difficult to put a name to. It's perhaps independence, however loving the family background, which mine was and still is. But there's perhaps more to it, something which I'm at a loss to name. Adulthood, it seems, is a one-way door.

As my endless typing continued, something else occurred. I admit I had bridled at the thought of applying for some menial post. Perhaps it had shown in my attitude in my talks with the resettlement officer when he had made that suggestion. Was it for this that I had worked my way through two universities and a postgraduate training college, seven years in all, gaining a total of at least seven high awards? I had my ambitions set higher than becoming a filing clerk, if I could secure even that. Perhaps that's just my pride again, but is it truly unjustified? Somehow I don't think so. As a comparison, no-one who spends years building a home for himself is likely to be content with being compelled to live in its garden shed. But necessity, I'd found, was a truly harsh mistress.

And that something else? The resettlement officer had found no posts, menial or not, available. He had to ask me: Was I prepared to undergo a course of training in a college for the disabled? And I too had no choice but to accept. The course would begin in a matter of months. It was at least something.

****

Some time later, I found myself yet again standing at college doors. It was all so very familiar, yet this would be something new too. The course intended for me was business studies, a completely unfamiliar territory. Other students appeared, these evidently newcomers also. Why not join in with the crowd and see what lay ahead?

At the opening assembly, it became obvious just how new an experience this was set to be. Already in my thirties, and with memories of the relative freedom of university days behind me, I grew increasingly uneasy. This was, we were told, an essentially residential college. We were not to leave the grounds except for a few hours in the evenings. But we were to be sure to return by a given time. We could return to our homes, but only at weekends. Buses would be available on Friday afternoon, but we must return under our own steam by Sunday evening. Otherwise, we were to consider the college premises our place of residence. Accommodation, at the time, was four to a room.

As these details were listed, my mind drifted to my father's description of National Service, three decades earlier. I couldn't prevent myself wondering what the consequences would be of failing to return on Sundays, as instructed. Would the offender perhaps be put on a charge, as my father, when serving as a non-commissioned officer, had sometimes done with conscripts? It was, I knew, a ridiculous notion, but one I couldn't remove from my mind. What we had just been told verged on the discipline of the barrack-square. Yet so it must be. We had no choice but to accept it. We were indeed now an army – an army of the disabled, as general society had labelled us.

Now it was time for the details of the various courses to be announced. Compulsory for all, it shook me to hear, was remedial English, totally regardless of previous experience. Yet in the months before entering the college, what had I done but translate? I had worked most of my life with language, and had actually taught English and linguistics. One of the other students in the fresh intake had been a senior civil servant, who had been broken down by acute depression. There was plainly no doubting his fluency, in the spoken and the written word. Yet there was no exception for him either, or for anyone else. Placed under the same discipline was one student who, like the ex-civil servant, became a close friend. In his earlier life, he had been an Air Force Provost-Marshal, whose duty had been to enforce strict discipline on others, much as I had done in the classroom. Now, like me, he was to be subjected to something similar.

It was this sense of the bizarre, even the unreal, which, I am convinced, prevented outcry. Old dogs, evidently, were to be taught even their own old tricks, no matter how well they could still perform them. But at least there was more: I had, I gradually realised, a slight knowledge of business, from studies of stocks and shares in mathematics classes during schooldays. This awareness was to be greatly increased, including by use of the computer, a piece of equipment which I had never so much as seen before. Here at least was a novelty.

Memories of school, almost twenty years earlier, served me well for that year. Mathematics had been at the time one of my favourite subjects. It was only its application to commercial use that I found at first strange. Proportion, percentages etc: yes, I had come across these before in an education system that, mercifully, considered mathematical success vital.

The computer at first had me mystified. The symbols and code words of the BASIC 'language' then in use were practically meaningless. It was maddening, for I could use the keyboard skilfully, but make no sense of what appeared on the screen before me. There must be a meaning, a key, to it, but I had no idea what it was.

Weeks passed as I struggled with BASIC and its applications. One evening, as I was idly reading a magazine in my shared room, a notion began to creep into my mind. Hadn't I seen something not so very different in the past? But what was it, and where? Days went by, and this idea refused to leave me. If anything, it was growing in strength. Then, finally, I woke abnormally early, with the answer to the riddle already in my head. BASIC was simply an altered version of school algebra.

I wrote down on the magazine some of the algebra I had learned in schooldays and compared it, also written on the magazine's margins, with a piece of the BASIC that I remembered from the day before. They were a close match, easily close enough for me to put to use in computing classes. I still remember well my first use of this idea: using the algebra-BASIC hybrid to work out a problem with taxation levels. After this, the whole idea made more and more sense.

I wasn't alone in finding irksome the return home only at weekends, in effect only for a day. Was this more like National Service or even a prison sentence? There seemed to be elements of both. At least as maddening were the compulsory remedial English classes, which we had to attend, without exception. Day after day, we had to write down the correct spellings of twenty words and hand these to the class instructor for correction, the same words often recurring. I had last known something like this when I was ten years old, at least twenty years before. I could see that I wasn't alone in approaching boiling point in this matter. Disability and low educational achievement don't necessarily go hand in hand, but that did appear to be the assumption, and, I've long realised, still is – and not only in the college.

After some short time, the instructor began to provide lessons on correct grammar, reading from a school textbook. I had reached my limit at this point. Linguistics and language had been my fascination, and still were. This was my territory, my speciality. In class one morning, I finally found myself loudly correcting the textbook as the instructor read it out. No, this usage could not be accurate, nor could this, except in given circumstances. There were surely exceptions of one kind or another, and I took care in explaining these.

I willingly admit that I made myself the class nuisance in this way. However the inaccuracies even of the textbook grated on my ear beyond bearing. Time after time, I interrupted the lessons. I was simply unable to prevent myself. It became practically a daily event, for I found the textbook riddled with errors.

To be honest, startled as he was at first, the instructor took my interruptions in good part as a whole and, from time to time, I noticed him secretly noting down my remarks for future use. I believe that he enjoyed our verbal jousts as much as I did, while the rest of the class enjoyed the diversion. From time to time, I noticed my ex-civil servant classmate, depressed or not, smiling behind a cupped hand.

And I must give the college and its staff their due: the training was of a high standard as a whole. Kitchen and room staff were more than considerate. Occasionally, I found a package of sandwiches slipped into my hand when it was end of term, and I would be visiting my family, who lived at a considerable distance.

Yet, to paraphrase the proverb, ointment does have a tendency to attract a fly. In the second or third week of our training, we came across him, one of the instructors in book-keeping. We knew him immediately for what he was, from his opening words. He wasn't, he claimed, doing 'charity cases' (his words) any favour by teaching us. The reality was that the college was only a short drive from his home. It was convenient for him. Even for that, he continued, we should be grateful.

I had seen him, or rather others like him, so often before. It was they who had hardened my skin. No-one responded, perhaps out of shock at his sheer arrogance, or perhaps, like me, out of experience. Everyone, I'm sure, knew well that the word 'disabled' suggests weakness, and it's always weakness that attracts the bully. Here he was, standing before us now.

He didn't fall short of that description. As days passed, he would single out a particular victim whom he would criticise mercilessly. Then it was another, then another. A favourite of his was actually a young man with Down's syndrome. Time and again, I watched him stand over this easy victim, barracking him to the point of tears. While this was taking place scarcely two metres away from where I sat, something told me no good would come of intervening, yet. What he was clearly enjoying doing was neither acceptable educational nor even human practice. I despised myself for saying nothing, but somehow realised this wasn't the time to speak. That time would come, and I would know it then. Like it or not, until then I must restrain myself.

After some months, I found his considerable bulk towering over me. I was being accused, apparently, of some virtually impossible falsification of figure work in a class examination. To have done what he accused me of, I should have to have somehow crept behind his back in a crowded classroom to change numbers on my paper, with a differently coloured pen. Clearly, I had become his choice of victim.

Now, I realised, it was the time at last. Sooner than even appear to show him any respect by rising to my feet, I replied, still seated: That any of us was capable of making errors - that was, if any such error had truly been made. By 'any of us', I included the instructor himself. However, he should be aware that I was not prepared to have anyone, and certainly not him, question my veracity. I would appreciate it, therefore, if he himself would arrange a joint interview with the college principal, where we could discuss the matter on equal terms.

I had never really thought of how he would react when eventually confronted. However, I could never have imagined what actually did follow. His right hand flew to his heart and he staggered back, mumbling some words about his own claimed condition. No-one rose to help him. He, now clearly a 'charity case' himself, would receive the same consideration as he had shown others. Besides, from past training in first aid, I could recognise this for the ham-acted pretence which it was.

Noticing how little regard his absurd charade was winning him, he achieved a remarkably quick recovery. Within minutes, he left the classroom and returned to provide me the details of our joint interview, in a few days to come. I readily agreed to attend with him, so as to settle matters. The class was dismissed early. Now, I realised, I could feel at ease with myself, whatever the interview might bring.

On the day set for our interview, I arrived early and sat outside the principal's office. No-one else appeared. At last, with only minutes to spare, the instructor arrived. Again, I remained seated. Was I really going to attend the interview? he asked, standing at my side. But of course, I replied, surprised. He had arranged it, at my request. Not to attend would obviously amount to insolence, at least to the principal.

He turned away again, and walked off down the corridor, leaving me to attend the interview alone. Rather than discuss the matter, I simply made a formal complaint about the instructor's behaviour, nodding towards the empty seat made available for him. To the reply received, that he was possibly doing only what was necessary to make unwilling students do their best, I suggested that perhaps he was over-playing his role. It seemed strange that no other instructor found adopting such an attitude necessary. Little more was said.

From then, the instructor's classroom manner was considerably subdued. He knew, I'm

81

convinced, that he had been shown to be the coward that, in reality, a bully invariably is. A coward fears nothing more than having his cowardice exposed, and most of all to his victims.

I have no idea whether he was ever disciplined following my complaints. That really matters very little as far as I am concerned, just so long as his behaviour was more moderate than it had been. Despite invitations from other staff members in later years, I've never visited the college again, something that still saddens me. I had my reasons: on the retirement of the original principal, it was that very instructor who was appointed in his place. I have no intention of meeting him again, and have nothing more to say to him. A less suitable head of a college for disabled people, for whom he had shown open contempt, I find myself unable to imagine. He was nothing more than the disablement officer whom I had rejected some years earlier. If he could show that open contempt for disabled people, then he himself deserved no better.

A bill may be slow in arriving, but any price must always be paid. It's a simple lesson in life which instructors, like anyone else, must learn. For treating disabled students as somehow lesser beings, he too had been forced to taste those same bitter cherries. For serving them to him, I haven't the slightest regret. If I have any regret at all, it's only that the opportunity hadn't come earlier. Experience had hardened me, but any bitterness must apply only to the cherries. This was my own simple lesson.

9: RETURN TO THE REAL WORLD

At the close of retraining, I was awarded a range of certificates, granted by various external, reputable examining boards. Among them were papers testifying to my ability to handle commercial mathematics, with credit, at all three levels, including advanced. My certificate for use of English showed a percentage well above ninety. Having finally mastered BASIC, I held another certificate for the use of the computer in business environments. Departing trainees, of whom I was one, were given the impression at least that our new skills would have prospective employers practically clamouring for our services. I, however, felt a degree of scepticism, for I had heard similar words in past years. My experiences didn't sit well with such optimism. Nonetheless, I could congratulate myself on completing yet another hurdle race.

My doubts proved justified, more and more as time passed. My applications even for minor office posts, running into several hundred in a further four years, usually received no reply. Applications for interview made by telephone, in the presence of the disability officer himself, regularly had the telephone placed down once my condition was mentioned. No other consideration seemed to matter. Still, at least these telephoned applications were dealt with immediately and did nothing to raise my hopes, unlike the written forms, which might just, in time, receive a positive reply of some kind, even invitation to interview. Few did.

Most application forms, I found, seemed almost designed to exclude anyone in my situation. Directly after the opening details, usually question four, came a request for information on any medical conditions. I had no choice but to disclose my epilepsy, although I took care to add that (as was the truth at the time) it caused me no real difficulty, in life or in work.

Then, in questions six or seven, came requests about previous employment, and reasons for leaving any posts held. My only ground for leaving earlier positions had been not my epilepsy itself, but others' attitudes and reactions to it. But if others had found me at all objectionable, for whatever vague reason, why would a prospective new employer risk taking me on his staff? In the final section of the forms, asking for additional information, or in supplementary letters, I did whatever I could to make my case. I had to appear to contradict myself, yet still seem convincing. For this reason, to complete a single form took hours, even days, of verbal gymnastics, leaving me exhausted and dispirited. Which made more sense: to prepare myself to hope, or steel myself for failure? I became increasingly skilled in the latter, if only out of experience.

However, there was no other choice but to try my utmost to prove simultaneously that, so to speak, two and two both did and didn't add up to four. My situation, I increasingly came to think, was at least a match for Heller's *Catch 22*. At times, in my imagination, I saw myself trying to play chess in three dimensions, but without knowing the rules familiar to my opponent. It was a ludicrous notion, of course, but it suited my dark humour at that time. I had to remain humorous, even in a strange way. The only choice was despair.

There was yet another difficulty. Certainly my new vocational qualifications were of value, and had been difficult to gain. However, I was forced to state that they had been won at a college for disabled people. Disability was not a popular term, and little understood, then or even in the present day. A survey taken twelve years after the eventual passing into law of the Disability Discrimination Act (1995) proved that, for a high proportion of the British population, quite what 'disability' meant still left them perplexed. They would be prepared, for example, to accept as a disability – that is, a lack of ability to carry out at least some everyday activities – the use of a wheelchair or a white cane. Many, however, considered people who find such aids necessary actually inconvenient, even distasteful.

Yet, to look at the other side of the picture, surely it's the disabled person who finds his condition genuinely inconvenient, and very much not to his liking. There seemed to be very few people in the survey who stopped to think of that side of the matter. Disability, hardly a deliberate choice, is and always will be an aspect of reality, to the able-bodied also. Remaining 'normal' is never certain; it can take no more than a sudden accident to change the 'normal' person's world, perhaps for life. Or, like me, he might wake one morning convulsing, for no obvious reason. Anyone can develop epilepsy at any time. Every year, many people actually do.

There was, however, less agreement about the less obvious conditions. Is, say, schizophrenia a disability? And is deafness? Plainly these are, but a high proportion of the public seem unconvinced, even yet. Psychiatric conditions of any kind were viewed with particular disapproval. About fifty per cent of those surveyed would feel uncomfortable, for whatever obscure reason, about even having a deaf person as a neighbour. It's scarcely surprising that wherever there's ignorance or confusion, prejudice can soon appear. Conversely, however, what percentage of disabled people would willingly have an able-bodied, but intolerant, neighbour? I suspect the figure would be well over fifty per cent.

Especially suspect were, and still are, people with 'covert' disabilities. And in this group, epilepsy figures highly. It's too simple, its doubters seem to believe, to feign attacks, and so 'sponge' on the state, whether or not the person with the condition had himself contributed to the state - when he could, and as I had done. Awareness of the true level of state benefits is too often grossly exaggerated.

In reality, it would be next to impossible for anyone to pretend to have a seizure, especially once medical help was summoned. The condition has too many features of which even the person experiencing the attack is usually unaware. This largely contributes to the difficulty of providing a description of the experience.

As another illustration of ignorance of the reality of disability, I've even heard broadcasters actually deny the existence of clinical depression, never mind the evidence. Yet I had seen it overwhelming my civil servant fellow student, not to say my ex-wife, almost to the point of breaking. It's widely recognised, unsurprisingly, as a cause of suicide. I knew very well that to dwell for more time than absolutely necessary on the attitudes displayed towards my own condition could easily cause such feelings in me too. It's a way of thinking I still practise, and strongly recommend.

Luckily, I had my books at home, which helped to turn my attention from other people's negativity and their rejection after rejection of me. I simply had to think of something else whenever I could. Eventually, I did receive psychological assistance, not so much for my epilepsy itself but to help with the scarring left by so many others' negative, often cruel, responses to it over the years. Anyone can cope only so far.

Still, there were some interviews, if only a few, following my intricately worded applications. Here, I repeatedly encountered what I've come to call the Tiny Tim concept, from the character in Dickens' *A Christmas Carol*. Interviewers, time and again, clearly struggled to grasp that someone who was disabled could be both mobile, without a wheelchair, and, more disturbingly still, highly qualified, sometimes to beyond their own level.

This plainly left them disconcerted. It challenged their stereotype. Why, I was asked repeatedly, was I applying for a low-level post for which I was clearly over-qualified? My reply, that only this was what might be available, had no effect. So much, it became obvious, for the resettlement officer's advice to 'take' a menial position. We can't take what isn't on offer to us. He had advised me, I remembered, to set out my goods, so to speak, on my market stall, prominently displayed. But what if I found my metaphorical stall continually kicked over?

It was becoming increasingly obvious that my compliant, open, approach was of little or no value. I would have to adopt, I realised, a more frontal assault technique, but at a time of my own choosing. In reality, there was no alternative. It might make me seem over-assertive, even arrogant. But what was the choice?

Eventually, I hit on the strategy of leaving out any mention of epilepsy on my application forms. Interviews multiplied, and I found myself offered attractive posts. It was only then that I mentioned my condition. Without fail, the offer was retracted. But, I had to ask, if I had been acceptable until that moment, how could I not be now? The interviewer knew what I had to offer him. Why should a minor condition like mine change my position? To my query, I rarely received a reply. An interviewer, once put on the spot in this way, seemed to have nothing to say to justify his changed stance. The reality of the situation was obvious: he didn't have a reason, only a vague fear of what epilepsy might possibly be, not the reality.

At times, I'd have preferred not to receive a reply. Some interviewers insisted as a condition of my employment that I would never have attacks during working hours. I had to ask, did they insist that other employees wouldn't suffer headaches in their working day? Headaches, I reminded them, didn't come at the times of our choice (if only they did!), and in just the same way neither did my attacks. One interviewer insisted on that same undertaking in writing. I had nothing more to say to anyone such as him and just left the room without comment. My expression, I still hope, made my feelings clear, for I had no words to express them. I still don't have them, so many years later. Any such undertaking would probably have been unenforceable in any case. However, I can see no point in investigating the matter. It doesn't seem to be worth the effort.

Another potential employer produced the most nonsensical response that I had heard. He would willingly, he claimed, make use of my services, but for (as always) my condition. No, he wasn't concerned that it would affect my performance; it was just that his first aid staff, when they had witnessed a seizure in the past, had been left demoralised, for at least the rest of the day.

I was staggered. Seeing a seizure left them 'demoralised'? What if a real emergency occurred, like fire or a serious accident? Perhaps that would demoralise them too? If so, he had obviously hired the wrong first aid staff, for they too would need first aid. That must surely be clear, even to him. Views such as his, I stressed, might well leave me demoralised – if I would allow them to. And that was a mistake I would never make. He could make of that whatever he wished. If anything was evident, his comments were nothing but yet another smokescreen against my disability. At least, some time later, I found them actually comical, something to smile at over my coffee.

And then there was another interviewer, who actually insisted that I demonstrate an epileptic fit in his presence. I could barely believe what I had just heard. If it were even possible, which it largely isn't, for someone to demonstrate an attack, to insist that I do so was demeaning at best, and showed the depth of ignorance present in this man. What did he want me to do? Should I perhaps roll on his office floor for a minute or two? There was nothing for it but to return fire, for this was too much by far. By all means, I replied with mock civility, I would do my best, but on one condition: that he should demonstrate to me the effects of a hangover. The intended outrage which followed my demand was, I willingly admit, deeply satisfactory as I stood up and left. One ignoramus had himself been made to experience the effects of demeaning talk like his own. In that achievement, I still take great pride.

A common viewpoint of what's become known as the 'epileptic personality' is that it's characterised by moodiness and irritability and a tendency to be reclusive. While there probably are some people with the condition who would have such natures in any event, in fact almost all of us find ourselves exposed over and again to ignorance and even contempt. Worst of all is a mixture of the two: an unwillingness on someone's part to be informed of the real truth of what the condition involves, for he can't be troubled to know. This is an attitude which I've encountered disturbingly often. We can't really be blamed then, I believe, if we tend to be on our guard more than many others.

To be fair to all, however, it is possible for someone to appear isolated, even uncivil, simply as a temporary side effect of medication for his condition. This was especially true, and generally longer-lived, with crude medications in the past. Even now, moodiness or even irritability can be a consequence of a change of medication. I've experienced these attitudes in myself, but only for a relatively short period, after the introduction of a new, greatly helpful medication. For almost two months, however, my letters even to friends sometimes verged on completely unprovoked insult. I discovered from the medication's insert that increased irritability was in fact a well documented, but temporary, reaction to the prescribed drug.

Much as I had enjoyed that achievement of demeaning my demeaner, it was still a brutal fact that I was going nowhere in finding work by any conventional method. I might despise the stereotype, as I did, of disability, but perhaps to make some concessions to it might have some effect. The disabled, I knew, were widely seen as achieving little in life. And so, I began to remove any mention not just of my condition, but also of my achievements, in application forms. My time spent in retraining was transformed into a period of unemployment. Out of interest, I pretended that my two years as a research student had been a spell of probation for some minor, unspecified offence.

Almost incredibly, an offer of interview followed shortly.

And again, positive replies to my applications multiplied. It was only when some, usually minor, post was being offered or was plainly about to be offered, that I told the reality, of both my condition and my achievements. Offers were instantly withdrawn. For showing the stereotype to be as hollow and meaningless as it was, I was anything but welcome. As far as I was concerned, that feeling was readily mutual towards many of my interviewers.

It remained in any case a fact that it was highly likely that a check on my background and references would reveal the truth to any deceived employer. The consequence could be that I would be branded as untrustworthy. Yet I knew well that to tell the truth too often made me unacceptable. I had no other option but to lie, for a dilemma on anything like this scale required extreme measures. And these measures, quite plainly, included lying and deceit when necessary, as it painfully often was. At least for some time, I might earn a living. For lying in this way, I still believe that I was completely justified and make no apologies. What choice did I have?

Several times, in writing to my then Member of Parliament, I commented on the odd discrepancy that there was in UK law a Rehabilitation of Offenders Act (an area in which I've done some work myself), and had been for years, but that nothing of the kind existed for the disabled, who could hardly be blamed for their situation. He readily agreed, but it was only after many years, and much parliamentary wrangling, that any such provision was passed into law. However, the Disability Discrimination Act, passed years after the similar Americans with Disabilities Act, has been scarcely a total success, as I've already tried to describe. Much more clearly needs to be done, which leaves an obvious question: Who is to do it? Law can at least attempt to prevent negative actions, but not the attitudes which underlie them.

I had spent a year retraining in a new area, business studies, no doubt at considerable public cost, and certainly with great effort. Yet my financial abilities have never been used in employment, however much I offered them. I've kept them, as a result, for my household budgeting or to help family or friends when requested.

10: THE BIG BREAK

Despite what had been trumpeted when I had won my vocational qualifications, finding work, at any level, was no different in the two years following my leaving the college from when I had first appeared at its gates. If anything, I noticed the difficulty had grown. For reasons I just can't understand, even now, British employers tend to be ill at ease when presented with what should surely be highly desirable and plainly very useful qualifications, and above all when a disabled applicant holds them.

Besides my keyboard and financial skills, I had command of several languages. Yet, at interviews (when I was granted any), employers tended to recoil. 'Over-qualification' and 'lack of job satisfaction' were their almost inevitable mantra. But wasn't that for me to decide? Would I consciously apply for work which I thought wouldn't satisfy me – just so long as I could perform to work specification?

And wouldn't advanced qualifications be a potential advantage to an employer? If my abilities went unused at first, wouldn't it be valuable to know that he had an employee already whose capacities could be utilised immediately, rather than having to fund an expensive recruitment process in future? I received no rational reply to these questions – in fact rarely a reply of any kind at all. It was plain that my background made me seen as a troubling anomaly.

Time after time, I found employers fastening on my health condition as a pretext for their twisted logic. When claims were made of its likely effect if I were taken on the staff, claims varying from insult to the absurd, I questioned deeper and commonly made a point of outstaying my intended time in the interview room. If this or that objection was made, I deliberately argued the point at length, if only to demonstrate my own abilities and to expose to the interviewer the hollowness of his alleged fears.

The employer's insurance premia would need to be raised? No that was untrue, even then. Shouldn't we consult together the terms of his liability certificate to check on that possibility? My suggestion was never granted. Potential colleagues might be disturbed by my presence and refuse to accept me? Not greatly long before, the same claim had been made about coloured people. However, that discrimination was now illegal and work colleagues, and potential employers, had been forced, however unwillingly, into line. How was I different? Would he please explain his viewpoint in some sensible, rational way? If he would, I was prepared to listen.

Yes, at these times, I was occasionally deliberately provocative, disrupting interviews in which I knew I had no hope in any case. There was no other way to leave my mark and, by discussion, to demonstrate that disabled people like me could hold their own. We weren't, and aren't, pathetic inferiors. If doing so caused my interviewer embarrassment, so much the better, for that was a clear sign that I'd won the argument. Let him brood on what I'd said, for I'd shown him a method of avoiding further pain in future.

It was the very same method I had used with students who had presented me with unsatisfactory, plainly careless, assignments. It was quite possible that I was gaining a reputation with interviewers. But what difference would that make, if I was likely to be met with rejection in any case? If I were treated with fairness, then I would respond favourably. That was my only condition.

I admit that my conduct of these interviews may sound aggressive or disaffected. Yet would that be at all unjustified? In actual fact, I was doing no more than forcing my interviewer to follow his logic, or lack of it, through. It was the way in which I'd been trained to think myself, and still do − and had taught others to do in previous years. On occasion it still causes annoyance, but there's no better weapon than persistent questioning against block-headed stereotyping and outright prejudice. I was being exposed to both. Why should I tolerate them? I hope that in explaining my way of thinking, I can do something to increase understanding of the aggression and irritability still often attributed to the 'epileptic personality'. If we're met with negativity, even hostility, how else can we respond? Yet what probably seemed like such aggression in me was, in reality, no different from the close, logical questioning of the courtroom.

Yet I was scarcely surprised by such events, for it was no more than I knew well from earlier experience. Not surprised by any means, but determined not to remain a passive target. I could return missiles, not just take them. If the original thrower felt some pain, the solution to his difficulty lay in his own hands. What I wasn't advocating was 'positive discrimination', for I regard this practice as patronising, practically as insulting as the negative variety. And so my application forms began again to bristle with my achievements – and my condition was mentioned. All details were given – and no interviews followed.

****

It's an odd phenomenon, one that I'm sure we're all familiar with, that a long-lasting problem in life can be solved practically and unexpectedly on the turn of a coin. Over years, I had applied for vacancy after vacancy, without results. I had changed my tactics to match my interviewers' own. I had no choice in the matter. Experience had taught me it was that or nothing.

After some more years of unemployment, I found one vacancy advertised, for a clerical assistant, in the local university. With CV in hand, but no real hope, I went along for what I was convinced would be the usual interrogation on my state of health. A young neighbour, glowing with pride in his recently-passed driving test, insisted on driving me the six miles or so there.

This was to prove something very different from before, anything but what I'd expected. In the interview room, with the head of the Department of Education, my health condition was practically waved aside. I was to begin not as a clerical assistant, but as a researcher soon, actual duties to be made clear at the time. Sadly, it was a short-term contract only, but the lack of insistence on my epilepsy left me bemused. What could I say when what couldn't happen had just happened? I must have been just staring, not quite sure of where I was. Awareness of success after so many years of failure had produced something not greatly different, if at all, from shock.

How had I travelled there? I was asked further. For refund of fares? I wondered. There hadn't been any, I stammered. A neighbour had driven me. So much the better, I was told. When I left, please send him in. The neighbour, in his late teens at the time, had never before been in a university. He passed through the door of the interview room petrified, as if to the dock of the High Court for sentence. Minutes later, he emerged. No sentence this: he had just been appointed my assistant. This was his first paid work. He said no more than that, clearly in a dazed state himself.

He drove me home again, both of us totally wordless. Had today really happened? Impossible. Reality would strike us soon. But this was reality. Letters confirming the appointments followed a few days later. A month or two later, I found myself on the research staff. This was an environment I knew well, one where I could flourish.

Duties were varied. Mainly, I was to compile a guide to historical research, complete with summaries. This, like Topsy, just 'growed and growed' over the months to follow, to at least 1,500 titles. I was seconded to libraries outside, to arrange old libraries, much of their contents centuries old and often composed in Latin. These documents too were to be summarised on index cards. But I was now making use of my abilities, no longer having to hide them, as previously. Reading documents composed in the handwriting of the 1600s or even 1500s, before they could even be translated, was no mean struggle, but not one where I'd had no past experience.

Another duty to be carried out was to interview and compile reports on overseas immigrants to the area, not by any means hostile reports, but only their impressions of life in a different country. This was a task, I was informed, for which my own living abroad, in the 1960s, seemed to suit me well. Almost without exception, these were people I came to respect deeply for their efforts to accommodate themselves to a greatly different way of life from that familiar to them. I can only hope that the impression which I left on them was favourable. That many later contributed to buy an ikon for my Name Day, painted on olive wood, at least seems to suggest so. And to be presented with this by a local overseas dignitary, before a group or seventy or so, and entirely without warning, was both a humbling and uplifting experience, one which I won't forget. That ikon, which I treasure for the positive view of me which those people took, still hangs on my bedroom wall.

For the first time in many years, I realised, I could now arrange an overseas holiday. Only a few years ago, it could have been so different. It would have taken so little. But best not to dwell on that. I must live now in the present and with what was, not with what might have been.

I returned invigorated, faced with new duties. With others, I was to compile reports on various aspects of local history, a long-forgotten group of (strangely enough) German swordsmiths and disused lead mine working, among others. It was thought-provoking, to say the least, to find the lead mining area surrounded by the graves of those who had worked there in the previous century. Many had been no more than children, who had carried out much of the refinement of the lead ore extracted from the seams in the hills, only to fall victims to lead poisoning or simple exhaustion.

This assignment meant visits in working hours to the appropriate sites. And all the time, the listing of historical theses continued to grow. It was an irony that most of the relevant material was housed in the historical library, practically in sight of the school which had disposed of me in such an inept way, and with such disastrous consequences. All of this too was something which I simply had to put behind me, however difficult. It was long over. Why dwell on it now? Yet how could I totally forget such an incident?

It was these reports, and the historical theses list, that led to a suggestion from my Department

Head. Why not produce, on my own account, a piece of work on the early history of the district? The idea touched something very familiar in me. This I knew well, and would do well.

Not greatly long later, I found myself called out to the Education Department on a Saturday morning. It wasn't for extra duties, but to attend a book signing. The university and the then EEC had reached an agreement to publish my short study of the early archaeology of the region. Yet only a few years before..... that thought wouldn't completely leave my mind.

I found ringing through my head that sunny morning, standing there in the Department hallway behind a pile of copies of my book with pen in hand, the old folk-tune: *The World Turned Upside-Down*.

What had happened so suddenly? It was impossible to grasp for a long time to come. In the event, my archaeological guide went into a second, enlarged edition. Sections were adapted for use in further local history studies. In time too, my historical theses guide was completed and handed over for publication.

Yet a short-term contract meant what it said. There was no prospect of extension. A year after my appointment, I left the Department for the last time. It was with regret, by all means, but I was heartened even so. I had found a fair employer, one prepared to take me at my own proven value rather than concentrating on one relatively trivial aspect of me. I owe much to those employers. It was largely thanks to them that I avoided deep cynicism, a characteristic which only too easily can develop into the poison of bitterness. Acceptance was, after all, a possibility. How could I not now be left in positive, uplifted spirits?

Yet the bluest of skies can show even a little cloud. After five years of separation from a wife I hadn't even seen in that entire time, I was forced to the conclusion that divorce was inevitable and set proceedings in motion, using legal aid. We would both at least have our freedom. After an interview or two with a solicitor, matters went ahead. I heard little more of the matter.

I was walking contentedly home from my workplace late one warm afternoon when I came across the solicitor in the street for the first time since our interviews the previous year. He was surprised, he remarked, since I plainly took the matter so seriously, that I hadn't attended the court hearing about ten days earlier. The divorce had gone through practically on the nod. I could expect the documents shortly.

There was the best of reasons that I hadn't attended, I replied: no-one had troubled to forward to me notice of the hearing. It would have been hurtful to be present at the close of the matter, as I had been present at the beginning, but it would have been altogether better in the long run. I had been denied even that, perhaps through some official's inefficiency. Perhaps someone had thought it not worth his while? Neither party, then, had been present at the hearing, however cursory it might have been.

I was divorced now, for over a week, and no-one had troubled to keep me informed? Somehow, I found this almost as shocking as the original break-up. When the documents did arrive, I read through them once and just put them away in a private place. I haven't read them again in more than twenty years. To read them again would just, I know, renew the hurt of that day. Over the years, I've mellowed. What had gone wrong was, I'm sure, nothing but a clerical error, not the result of malice of any kind. Yet such a mistake at such a time! Deliberate or not, it hurt deeply.

The search for my now ex-wife had produced no results. No-one could find her whereabouts. Did she ever receive copies of the divorce papers? Did she regain her health? Did she ever find happiness with some new partner, somewhere? Was she by then even alive or dead? To all of these questions, I still have no reply. It was in its own way like what I had found some time after the break-up: all photographs which showed either her or me, or both, had been carefully removed from albums while I was absent from our home. She had simply disappeared from the scene, totally, and I too had been erased from the history of the past six years. It couldn't have been more final, even at the beginning of the break-up.

There had been a parallel of a kind in my earlier life. Another researcher at my earlier university, working in the same department, had become increasingly uneasy as his student visa was reaching its end. Efforts to renew it failed. He could foresee only too clearly the likely future of his home country, Chile, to which he had no choice but to return in 1973, the very year when a military junta seized power. For some short time, we had corresponded, but only for a year or so. After then, my letters to him had been returned unopened. Did he simply lose my address, or change his own, forgetting to inform me? In one way or another, he had simply disappeared from the scene.

Perhaps ominously for us, his last piece of correspondence had been a congratulations card on our marriage. What has become of either person I still have no idea, many years later. For both I can only wish the best, and try not to fear the worst. Perhaps it had been political upheavals which had led to the loss of my ex-colleague, perhaps not. The cause of the loss of my now ex-wife and so much more was only too plain. It was a single, but deeply significant, word: epilepsy. Only a few letters long, yet in the document long before demanding my disbarment from education, it had actually been misspelled.

11: PUSHING THE ROCK

A year of accomplishment behind me, and a highly enjoyable one at that, even if there had been a painful development in connection with our divorce – but the old question arose, as ever. What now? Back to searching for work: it seemed to be my fate, like rolling the mythological rock uphill just to weary when I was a footstep short of the summit – and watch the rock roll downhill again.

If there was one thing, I had decided, I would never do again, it would be to hide my light under the proverbial bushel. No, like before, I would go on the offensive. Sooner do that than meekly tolerate someone else's offensiveness. There had been quite enough of that in the past. There would be no more meekness, no more effacing myself. Why should I? Application forms were completed, but with all achievements described – and, yes, my condition mentioned, making as little of it as it deserved. And that, in reality, was almost nothing, if anyone was prepared to listen. Surely my listed details on the form made that clear? But no, they didn't. I was too used to this by now to feel remotely frustrated, only bemused. It was long obvious that there were no marks granted for trying, even having succeeded against the odds.

On the rare interviews which I did secure, I made a point of pressing that point home, that my condition hadn't stopped me, however long it might take to make my interviewer, exasperated or not, see sense. There was no reason why my condition should stop me now, was there? What had stood in my way, and still did stand there, was just a single, simple word. Yet in terms of success, it might as well have been the inscription above the door to the Inferno: Abandon Hope. But that I wouldn't do. It didn't matter if I argued my interviewers to a standstill, especially when it was plain that I had not the slightest chance of success anyway. If anything, those were the times when I argued hardest. Why not hit hard, when I had nothing to lose? As someone said long ago: let the die be cast.

I still think of these, with a smile, as my kamikaze applications and interviews. I might well go there, as I did, but had little or no chance of returning with anything like success. Still, I would have made my point. More and more I was content with that. I had no real choice. Now that I can think back to those days, I realise that the truth, however unfair it might be – and was - had begun to dawn. I was prepared to argue at such length, and felt no disappointment when the rejection letter arrived, as it only rarely did. Usually there was no reply. It now troubled me not at all. I had done my best, and could deserve to heat myself another coffee, sitting in my kitchen. One important thing remained: I must have something to read.

I'm aware now why I gradually felt this way. The only person who can feel disappointment is the person who has hope to begin with. Still, I remained prepared at least to try, even if I knew well that the very few letters which followed would be barely worth the effort of cutting them open. This wasn't negativity, but a realisation of what appeared, for some unknown reason, inevitable. Before and after interviews, I no longer lay awake at night rehearsing and revisiting my arguments and self-presentation. They had become all too familiar. I could sleep in peace – and did. And I still do. It was, and still is, enough to have tried. What more could I do?

However much I might highlight my past, and very recent, achievements, there was one thing I knew I mustn't mention: that I had a published book, now in its second edition, to my name. I was too familiar by now with what was seemingly the endemic philistinism of too many British employers. They were distrustful enough of someone who had read books. The very thought that the person they might be interviewing had actually written one! I had actually had better success when I pretended I had been on a period of probation. I still can't understand this mentality. Was it somehow more normal, or even acceptable, for someone to have fallen foul of the law? That's what I didn't want to believe, but my experience seemed to indicate. If I wanted work, it seemed better to serve a sentence than to write one.

Two years of this absurdity trailed on and on. If anyone despaired, it was the disability resettlement officer. I didn't, for my skin had long since hardened too much for that. In time, the officer cast his last, desperate throw: I might go for further training, again.

I can't express highly enough just how much I value achievement and accomplishment, which involves training of some kind, and above all for disabled people. Nothing shakes the stereotype more, which was and remains a major part of the problem. Regardless of any evidence to the contrary, too many others preferred the stereotype. And that baseless stereotype of disability had, and still has, to be broken.

I couldn't help wondering as the disability officer made his suggestion. Each time I had taken up training, it was with the idea that this way I might seem more desirable to an employer. But no, more and more I found myself trapped in a fog of 'over-qualification', whatever that might be. Perhaps it's significant that I find this term only in English. I'm familiar with a range of languages, and can't translate it into any of them. It seems to be a notion lurking only in the brain of the English-speaking interviewer. How was it even thinkable that I could escape from the 'over-qualification' trap by gaining more qualifications? It seemed, in one of my more detached moments, like handing to a condemned man a spare rope, just in case something went wrong (or right, depending on viewpoint.) To maintain my sanity, I had to keep my humour, however grim it might seem at the time. Whatever the saying, that in the country of the blind even the one-eyed man is king, the truth of the matter was very much the opposite.

And what was the further training suggested to me this time? I could try my hand, the officer suggested, at word-processing, something I knew nothing about and had scarcely heard of at the time. Still, I would show willing and, in any case, I would collect a few pounds weekly above basic benefit levels just for attending the course. Training would begin at a college near my home, thankfully this time not residential. And it was at this college that I appeared some time later.

It has to be admitted that word-processing, once I had grasped the idea, took my fancy. I was already familiar with the typewriter keyboard, so adjusting to the more elaborate keyboard took little out of me. The ideas expressed in the handbook made more and more sense by the day. Paperless typing had much to recommend it.

This, however, was only part of my training. Far more time was spent in an increasingly interesting area. I was assigned to the unit which produced magazines for the blind and virtually blind. This, I could see, was highly valuable, for I knew for myself the limitations that disability places on anyone.

It was an intriguing idea. A collection of daily newspapers appeared each morning. The most important or interesting material was collected, typed up in a different form and then read on to a bank of audio-tapes. At the end of the week, these were sent off by the hundred to registered blind people throughout the country, with a request for their return for re-use the following week and, in particular, comments on the content and suggestions for improvement. Most were returned, usually with compliments, but in the way of things some we never saw again. There were rumours later,

I believe probably accurate, that some of these had found their way to the US or Canada, even Australia. I still think of this as a compliment, of sorts, an opinion shared by the six or so others in the unit. In quieter moments, I taught two or three of these the use of the QWERTY keyboard, in which they went on to gain qualifications.

However, as I'd found before, the retraining college had its apparently inevitable bully. There was no point, it was obvious, in complaining about him to the principal. He was the principal. It has to be said for him that he wasn't lacking in courage. Courage was his Alsatian dog which he kept by his side on its leash as he made his seemingly endless patrols of the college corridors.

We learned not to close doors fully shut, whatever the time of the year. The principal's management style was to throw open training room doors and glare, often wordlessly, as he strode indoors for a few minutes, or remove a newspaper. Him we treated with open indifference; it was his rather friendly Alsatian for which we reserved our smiles as she stood there cheerfully wagging her tail. Even Courage, however, came at her price, if a small one. From time to time, our recording sessions were interrupted by her distant barking. Back to the beginning, and the sessions recommenced with our fingers crossed for luck. It seemed at times almost surreal, but it was nothing with which all of us weren't well familiar before long.

The surreal became normality. In that building, it had to be. Since my background was known, an extra use was found for me in time, one which truly did pose a difficulty. Personal histories of trainees were collected and passed to me to recast into acceptable résumés for possible future employers. Certainly, this was familiar ground for me. However, now the picture was reversed. Almost without exception, the younger trainees had what would have been an astonishingly low level of attainment and literacy, startling except to an ex-teacher.

Their personal backgrounds were more of a problem. A high proportion had court convictions, not necessarily for minor offences. To rephrase these into what might seem attractive to a potential employer strained my diplomatic skills to the limit. Yet hadn't I done something not greatly different on my own behalf for years? My own experience was put that to full use. And, on and on, these histories appeared on my desk.

Over that year, I recast something over four hundred into what may have been at least potentially acceptable résumés. How was I to disguise fact, yet remain truthful – in a way? I had to find a way, just as I had done in writing up my own past applications. History after history presented some such problem. I returned to my past writing up of school report cards. Remarks there too had to hover, time and again, somewhere between positive suggestions and something not greatly short of offensive comments, even if well deserved. How many of my recastings were successful I was never informed, perhaps for the best. I could adjust or dress up the facts as told, but not change them.

It wasn't only trainees' details which found their way to me for rephrasing and typing. Instructors ambitious for new posts passed their applications to me for typing in some formal way. Here was a dilemma. A growing number of these applications showed a level of literacy scarcely higher, if at all, than those of the trainees. I found many riddled with grammatical and spelling errors for which I would have been shown no mercy as a schoolboy.

So what was I to do here? If I didn't correct the scripts, as my fingers itched to do, there was every chance that some of the repercussions of the applicants' failed interviews would be directed towards me. However, if I did correct them, wouldn't that be likely to cause insult – and bring more flak my way in any case?

Basic logic solved the difficulty. Anyone, I reasoned, who was capable of producing such a low standard of material would surely be unlikely to be aware that it had actually been corrected. All I had to do was leave the changes I made unmentioned and my troubles would be over, the problem solved. And this is precisely what happened. For one reason or another, various staff members vanished. What became of them, whether they were successful or not, I never knew. I considered that it might perhaps be better for me not even to ask. I had difficulties enough to deal with already. Why look for more?

Yet another duty was assigned to me: to collect material for the in-house magazine. Usually, this meant conducting interviews, something with which I was very familiar. I was to take the accompanying photographs too, for the only camera available was almost identical to my own, and only I apparently was familiar with its operation.

This was rewarding work. Staff and students alike: some had remarkable stories to tell, of past and present activities. One young female staff member, apparently a quiet and peaceful individual, turned out on interview to be a highly enthusiastic member of a group dedicated to recreating the conflicts of the mid-seventeenth century civil wars. I declined with thanks her invitation to join the group. I already carried quite enough scars on my body as a result of my blackouts and collapses. Adding to these even the possibility of strokes from blunted swords or blows from cannon barrels would be, even in my experience, stretching reality just that little bit too far.

Naturally enough, my seizures occurred as usual. Regular practice was to have me driven home almost immediately, when in fact a short recovery time was all that would be really needed. I have to admit that I didn't entirely object to this practice. Besides, it's reasonably common for an epileptic attack to be followed by an intense headache, lasting hours but only rarely overnight. Here I saw an advantage.

Occasionally, the morning after an onset, I would telephone the college with claims that the headache was continuing. It would be wise, they agreed, to stay at home. This settled, I promptly went outdoors to visit the real world. I reasoned, surely even Hieronymus Bosch, the Renaissance artist who specialised in painting imaginary scenes of

113

Hell, must have needed time from his duties, authorised or not. Why should different rules apply to me? The glaring, the audio-magazines, even Courage could wait their turn. Now I could steal a little time for myself. No-one would be the worse for my short absences and I would be all the better. It was surely only the sensible thing to do.

And the time finally came for my valedictory message on the audio-magazine, just as I wished my colleagues goodbye and walked home from the college for the last time. Some time later, I received by mail my certificate in word-processing, certifying a high level of proficiency. Experience had taught me its likely value in securing work: that it could easily make matters more difficult still. Nonetheless, it did gain a mention in future applications. Why not, when I had to undergo prolonged training to gain it? The certificate remains even now in my private papers, along with the many others gained.

Since I had left the educational world, practically none of the vocational qualifications I had won from them had been put to any practical use, except in my short spell as a research assistant. Now here was another. At least I felt the better for its arrival, whatever view others might take. By now, that scarcely seemed to matter.

12: GOODBYE TO ALL THAT

Whatever my other duties at the college, I pursued my training in word-processing. I knew that I must have something to offer when the time came to leave. And that something would have to impress, for on occasion I had found myself sent home during the day. There had to be something to counterbalance this problem.

Usually, but not always, unaware as I was of the occurrence of attacks, it nevertheless wasn't difficult to judge why this was being done, even though only a few minutes' recovery time would have been necessary. Were administrative staff concerned only with their own wellbeing and security?

This became a more and more unavoidable impression: that they saw me as a threat in some illogical way. If so, it was nothing new. Yet, some of those in the training centre, as I could see from their résumés, had been convicted of violent crime. These remained on site, while I was sent home, as if somehow more of a risk. Just where, I longed to ask anyone, was the sense in all this? Yet, in so many areas, it had been a feature of my life with epilepsy. Sense, logic and reason: all had disappeared from the scene. There was definitely in the atmosphere an aura of unease, almost fear. But why?

I had had a reasonably parallel experience from some years earlier. Once, while in a department store in a large city some distance away, I found a shop manager standing over me where I sat propped against railings a short way from the exit. Obviously, I'd briefly lost consciousness in an attack. I was to stay where I was, the manager said, while helping me to my feet. He had called for a taxi to take me home, even though I had clearly been about to leave anyway. The £10 note he pressed into my hand would cover my fare, he assured me. But why a taxi, I couldn't help wondering? If I seemed to him to need help at all, wouldn't an ambulance be more appropriate? But it was surely plain by now that I didn't need help. Why not cancel the taxi? There was no more need for it, if there ever had been. Wasn't that obvious to him, I protested?

I was twenty miles or more from home, but he wasn't to be gainsaid. Obviously, for I made my destination clear, the journey home by taxi cost considerably more - an amount to be supplemented from my miserly unemployment allowances. Epilepsy, I've often found, can be an extravagant condition, not one to be recommended.

Wouldn't it have been vastly simpler just to let me sit for some minutes and regain my breath? I was within sight of the store café, with its ranks of unoccupied seats. It was a point which I tried to make, only to find it brushed aside. It's occurred to me more and more over the years that the truth may well have been rather that I was seen as an embarrassment. Perhaps I gave the impression at first of being drunk, even though it must have almost immediately become obvious that this wasn't the case. Or did he think that it would be preferable for the public not to see me on the premises? By way of comparison, would he have stopped at the door anyone using a stick or a crutch, say?

I'll take, still with some difficulty, the more charitable view, that he had what he considered my best interests in mind, even if he did leave me heavily out of pocket. Regrettably, however, the other viewpoint remains a strong possibility. It chimes too closely with the disability officer's offer to me, years earlier, of an opportunity of work. But only, the potential employer insisted, if I was kept out of public view, for an attack, even slight, might perhaps cause some disturbance in customers.

Surely understandably, I'd refused this as an insult (and had been criticised for refusing.) Regardless of criticism, this is how I still think of that suggestion. I have my pride and self-respect too, as do others with disabilities. We aren't lesser people, only slightly different in one way or another from the average person. This is no reason to put pointless difficulties in our way. Nature has already done that, and we must learn to cope with them. There's no requirement for society, usually pointlessly, to repeat what nature has already done.

It was regular policy of the retraining centre, when trainees had completed their time there, to direct them into some position at least to start employment. Once, during my training, I had been called on, without warning, to act as an interpreter when instructors from a similar centre arrived from Germany. My linguistic background was well known, so what at least appeared to be an appropriate post was found for me.

This was in the offices of a specialist translator, dealing mainly with material to be translated from German. Day after day, I found

117

passed to my desk technical papers referring to engineering, for example the details of public transport and their driving mechanisms. Yet, while my father had been an engineer, I had myself, and it was well known, no background or expertise whatever in that area. As I struggled with these documents, I found myself wondering: did I understand them better before or after translation? The college's thinking when directing me to this post had been plainly simple, if not simplistic. I could deal with words; that must mean any words. But this isn't what translation is about. It deals with meaning, not just words. It was as plain to the translation agency's manager as it was to me: I was floundering, sinking slowly below the surface.

We agreed after only a week or two: I couldn't guarantee the accuracy of what I had been struggling to translate. There was no point in my staying there. I had to find another niche. It was a familiar situation, no longer even painful. No need to show me the door; I already knew where to find the exit, and left with deep relief, no doubt shared by the manager.

The close of my two years' training saw me presented with a posted certificate, again with merit, in word-processing. There was an offer also of an interview, as an office assistant at a security services company. Security services? Again, this was something I knew nothing about. Just possibly, however, my work with the résumés of so many trainees would provide me with background of some sort that might prove helpful.

When the day came for the interview, I told the truth of my condition and, very much to my surprise, found myself appointed nonetheless. The payment for a week's work was barely above unemployment benefit levels. I had to fund my own transport and pay for my own meals. Still, it was a beginning. I'd been accepted. Who was to say where that might lead? Ambition began to grow again, after its long hibernation.

The main duties of my post in the typing pool were to prepare outgoing correspondence and keep a check on personnel files. Here my earlier experiences in recasting résumés did come in very handy. With practice, it becomes a simple matter to notice when there are certain things an applicant prefers not to mention. It's difficult to describe: a mixture of certain key words and distortions in sentences. These were the applicants whose references had to be checked with particular care. Time and again, caution won out. Previous employers, when contacted, were only too pleased to dispense with these candidates' past services, commonly for unsavoury reasons. Then it was my duty to compose the rejection letters.

Strangely, school teaching experience proved valuable too. It doesn't take much practice for even a newly qualified teacher to decide when copying of work has been carried out, this or that detail somehow changed, or when homework genuinely has been accidentally left at home. These, and a multitude of other such sins, find their way into the industrial world too, even if in a rather different form.

My typed correspondence drew praise from the personnel manager. He was saved the tiresome duty, as he told me in person, of checking mail. He could now rely on it to be word-perfect. It was all the more important since, soon, the professional authorities would carry out a snap inspection. There was no questioning this, for the tension in the building was only too plain. That apart, things were looking up for me. In checking the personnel files one day, I came across my own file. Here I was described as showing great future potential. Nonetheless, I'd have preferred my colleagues to be more talkative than they were. Clearly, however, the strain of the oncoming check was reaching them too. This was only to be expected.

Six weeks or so after my appointment, the workplace tension had become almost overwhelming. A note arrived on my desk. The personnel manager would like to have a word with me in private at the lunch break. I was too experienced by now not to know perfectly well quite what this really meant, or really care very much. I was too used to it. The only question was what form it would take, something to think over idly while typing letter after letter as the day passed.

At lunchtime, I duly arrived at the personnel office and was invited to take a seat - the very seat, I remembered well, where I'd sat on the day when I was appointed. The personnel officer cleared his throat and half stammered:

"Look, this just isn't working."

"Isn't it?" I replied. "Why not?" It was no time, surely, since he'd complimented me on my standard of work, although I knew from painful experience this was no guarantee of anything. Sometimes it had been the very reverse: a smile with a threat. The raised dagger tended to follow.

It was what he had to say next which left me stunned. My work colleagues, I was told, were unwilling to work in my presence, out of concern for my attacks. But how could I possibly harm them? As for the growing tension and the surliness of my colleagues, the coming inspection had little connection with these. I was the cause, it now appeared, of the workplace stress, which had begun to provoke relatively minor attacks in me. Stress was causing attacks, and attacks were causing stress. It was an impossible cycle, one I knew painfully well.

The real refinement, however, had yet to come. One of my now ex-colleagues, apparently the sternest of them all, had expressed fear of being bitten during one of my attacks. Not a word had been said to me. I stared into his face, at what supposedly was a private interview, waiting for him to smile. Possibly he had mistaken my birthday date for some workplace prank? But smile was what he failed to do. I realised, incredulously, that he was speaking seriously. A nonsensical fear had been given precedence over my proven standards.

It was only a few years since I'd been dismissed on suspicion of perhaps being some form of human firebrand. Was I now being treated as

121

something akin to a vampire? How could anyone make such a claim and expect it to be taken seriously? Yet this was just what I could see before me. Each face I scanned in a slow circle was as serious and poker-faced as the next. No, I wasn't dreaming. This was entirely genuine. I was asked, with an attempt at civility, to leave at the end of the day.

As I rose, at my choosing, to leave the room, I considered my options. A vampire, we read, can wait for the fatal stake through the heart or, if he has any sense, make his exit at the first scent of garlic. I would be the sensible vampire. I wouldn't wait until the end of the week, or even the end of the day. I would go now, and leave my now ex-colleagues untroubled any longer. As for the paperwork on my desk, the sheet in the typewriter roller, someone else, no doubt without fangs, could deal with it in my place.

It was as I was making my way down the stairs that I met my youngest colleague, who had been sent on work experience from school. He had tried, he said, to calm the others when I had had one of my attacks, and to help me. Yet it had been impossible to prevent one in particular from running screaming from the room at such times. This was, from his description, perhaps the same person who had feared being bitten.

It's a strange phenomenon, one I can't understand. When anyone is prepared to keep his head and offer practical help during an epileptic attack, not only mine, it's almost without exception a young person. This still happens on occasion. I've commonly found myself helped by untroubled, younger people, the contents of my pockets untouched. What it is and when that makes the undisturbed young person become the disconcerted and distrusting adult is something I'd dearly love to know. Given the nature of the learning process, the development should surely be the very reverse, as a person gains knowledge and experience. Yet, for whatever reason, this isn't what happens in reality. I can't begin to guess why.

As I left the building, early that afternoon, into the June sunshine, I realised that this had to be an end, if only for my own sake. My original two daily tablets, only a low dosage, when the condition had first appeared, had now mushroomed into seventeen per day, not far short of toxicity. Attacks at first had been a rare occurrence, barely noticeable, if at all. I'd been aware for some time, and friends confirmed my suspicions, that with each struggle to find or keep work the attacks had only become more severe and persistent, sometimes several in series. It was obvious that I couldn't prejudice my own health and wellbeing any further. Add to that the losses sustained: career, home and marriage. No more taps on the back from a sickly-smiling manager, without warning, to inform me that leaving, and losing my livelihood, would be somehow all for my own good. It was over now. Twenty-two years of struggle to find and keep work, training and retraining yet again, were quite enough for anyone.

Strangely, as I slowly promenaded through the sunny streets down to the bus station, a great weight lifted from me and a memory returned from the distant past. It was only a short phrase from the national anthem of a South American republic: *abajo cadenas* ('Cast off your chains'). That was what I'd now done. Admittedly I had placed the chains on myself, in my attempts to conform to the 'normal' world, whatever that might be. However, I might expect the 'normal' world to reciprocate, and this it hadn't done. In my attempts to find a working life, I'd gathered around thirty certificates in a range of areas, most of a high standard, and awards, not to mention other achievements. They'd counted for nothing. At times, they'd even been held against me and I'd been forced to conceal them. I'd damaged my own health in my attempts to conform. The time for this, for biting my tongue under others' ignorance and even insults, and for arguing against absurd fears, was at an end. I'd done my best, and no-one could ask more, for there was no more to give.

No, I decided as I made my way slowly down the sunlit street, I wouldn't go straight home. That would be like running away, like escaping to my lair. Without purpose or destination, I simply walked through one street after another, bathing in the warmth and light. And only very gradually, from under the ashes of my past twenty years, I became aware of another warmth, now from within. My vital spark, however bleak the past, had never really died completely away. Now it was at my service, for my life was my own again.

The next working day, I finally gave in to the definition I had refused to accept for so many, often painful, years and had my name accepted on the register of those incapable of employment on ground of severe disability. Or was it perhaps more sensible to consider the 'normal' world I'd had to tackle as itself disabled in some strange way? It didn't really matter and still doesn't, for it wasn't my affair any longer.

APPENDIX

FIT FOR LIFE

A: TELLING IT LIKE IT IS:
THE FACTS OF LIVING WITH
EPILEPSY

Only occasionally, I'm asked what it's like to have epilepsy. I wish I were asked more often, for then I'd be able to spread more real information about this condition. It's surrounded by hopelessly outdated notions and assumptions, many dating back centuries or even longer. The only way to confront these is to provide the real truth of the matter, and best of all from someone who has it and so can speak from experience.

It isn't, however, an easy question to answer. There's no one description of the condition. It's very much an individual matter. To begin, let's take a look at the classic depiction of a seizure on film or on the stage:

Suddenly the person stares silently, staggers back and collapses, convulsing violently. Someone calls out 'It's epilepsy' and forces a stick into the mouth of the sufferer, whose jaw is by now rapidly opening and shutting again, over and over. After some minutes, the person with the seizure slowly rises to his feet, dazed and shaken.

It's understandable, up to a point, that epilepsy is often shown in this way, for graphic and dramatic reasons.   Even so, it strengthens some existing, mistaken notions about the condition. First, only about one in three or four epileptic attacks causes convulsive collapses (now called tonic-clonic seizures). Most don't do anything of the kind. It can easily happen for someone to have an attack in company, yet no-one else even notices. I've known this many times. My hearing or my vision (sometimes both) becomes confused, for example, for a few minutes, yet I can still behave perfectly normally and stay aware until the attack passes, for I do know what's taking place and how to deal with it - usually by just sitting down calmly until the attack passes over.   This, however, doesn't always apply. In over forty years I've had the violent, tonic-clonic sort of seizure on occasion, but only very rarely.

Secondly, it's often thought to be a consequence of injury to the head or illness.   It certainly can be, but in most instances – again in about three cases out of four – it has no known cause. At one stage or another in life, younger or older, it just appears and no-one knows why. This is idiopathic epilepsy, and my own condition is one such case. When I had my first seizures, at about fourteen, I was in the best of health otherwise and had certainly suffered no injuries to the head. Something of this sort often applies. It has no rhyme or reason, but suddenly makes itself known, whether or not there's a family history of the condition. I'm the only known case of epilepsy in my family, the reason that my first seizures caused such alarm. My family had no idea what was happening to me, and neither did I, that fateful first morning.

I suspect that the widespread idea that epilepsy always involves convulsions, when in fact only a small number of attacks do, is at least part of the reason that people in general tend to think of it as rare. The true number of cases is perhaps startling: in Britain alone, the figure for people who have had at least one attack is around 400,000. Persistent cases, like my own, reach, on present figures, about 250,000, and more are recorded daily. In the United States, there are well over two million such cases. We can only make an estimate of the figure for people with epilepsy worldwide. One suggestion is that it's more than forty million people. I suspect, however, that this figure is probably too low. Many, regrettably, of these people live without medication for the condition, for it isn't available where they live.

And one very wrong message given by the dramatic presentation is that the right approach is to force a walking stick or something similar between the jaws of someone having a convulsive seizure. In fact, this is one very likely way of damaging the person's teeth. If it's absolutely necessary, say to avoid the person biting his tongue, a soft object should be used to keep his jaws separate, with care taken to avoid suffocation and to prevent convulsive beating of the person's head against a floor or pavement. Something never to use to help in this

131

way is one's hand. I've actually heard people complain that, during the seizure, the person they had tried to help had bitten them. If so, it's hardly surprising, and it certainly wasn't a deliberate action. The person convulsing had very probably lost all awareness for some time.

It's probably surprising, too, to learn that there's more than one type of epilepsy. In fact, the true figure for the different varieties of the epilepsies is, at present, around forty. This is another reason that it can be such a difficult condition to describe. Most difficult to describe, since it can take so many forms, is perhaps what's thought to be the most common variety: temporal lobe epilepsy (TLE), which I have myself.

To explain a little, at least as far as I am able to: it's generally recognised that a human brain is the most complex, and still least understood, object known to humankind. It's divided into a variety of sections, or lobes, each, or with others, governing one aspect or another of our being. Some relate to hearing, to language, to vision or to behaviour. Vision, for example, is located in the rear of the skull. Light signals passing through the eyes focus on the retina, which passes them as an electrical signal to the visual area. It's only then that we can understand what we are seeing, almost instantaneously.

Reasoned, thoughtful behaviour is thought be governed in the brain area in the forehead. This is especially likely, however, to be influenced by alcohol, which is why someone who is drunk so often acts out of character.

The temporal lobes, just above and behind either ear, are still only partly understood. Among their other functions, they seem to deal with the emotions. They are an immensely complicated part of an immensely complex structure, the brain. And TLE is, as I've said, a particularly common, yet rarely mentioned, form of epilepsy. Finding the words to describe a TLE can be, even for an eloquent adult, sometimes next to impossible. A younger child may be left simply bewildered, without the words to describe his experience. No-one is likely to find it easy.

What causes epileptic attacks? In any particular seizure, slight or severe, some brain cells seem to misfire and to confuse the natural brain electricity (these misfires are identified on the electro-encephalograph, or EEG, as characteristic 'spikes' in brain activity). The effect of the misfires depends largely on where in the brain the disturbance takes place and how far it spreads.

Since the temporal lobes are so complex, a disturbance in these can take any number of forms. Sometimes my hearing is affected, leaving me in an otherwise quiet place surrounded by what appear to be pulsing, painful vibrations. Or it can be affecting my vision, so that colours reverse or disappear altogether. At other times, their intensity can grow. It's now believed that Van Gogh had a form of TLE, given his fascination with intensely bright yellow, as in sunflowers.

It sometimes even appears that I can see sound (an effect known as synaesthesia, when two or more senses become confused). On occasion, as I'm sitting in a café or a bus or train, the words of other people's conversations appear like silvery-blue flashes, like tracer bullets, aimed at the centre of my forehead. The longer it lasts, the more painful it becomes, even though I'm usually not concerned with what they're saying. Yet what I mustn't do is stand and move away. There's an increased chance that at these times, if I stand, I'll stagger or collapse. I can only sit and wait until it passes, usually after a few minutes.

Epilepsy – and not least TLE – often increases a person's sense of atmosphere, perhaps the reason that it's often associated with religious devotion. I commonly experience a form of *déjà vu,* or, more rarely, its very opposite, *jamais vu* (the sudden notion that I've lost all knowledge of even the most familiar people or places). I can sit at home, for example, and suddenly realise that I haven't the slightest idea of where I am or what day it is. What were, only minutes earlier, things I'd actually been using, I've suddenly never seen before. I don't know any longer even what they are.

Luckily, these spells rarely last more than a few minutes. After any attack, it's important, if it's at all possible, to stay seated for some short time. Attacks can occur in series. On at least one occasion, I've known twenty or more collapsing seizures, lasting for hours and leaving me severely injured, in my own bedroom. Its cause was

134

discovered shortly afterwards, once medical help came. A summer flu, so mild I wasn't even aware of it, had raised my body temperature just enough to cause the attacks. For this reason, any condition of this type, even the common cold, makes it wise for me to stay indoors, regardless of circumstances or my intended arrangements. Not doing so is a risk that's just not worth taking.

I have to avoid, too, lack of sleep and over-anxiety. This was in the past another paradox: that failing to find work made me increasingly anxious, which caused further attacks, and this discouraged employers from appointing me. Yet the security of employment would be likely to reduce any attacks. This exasperating double bind, however true it was, I found impossible to explain to interviewers. Even if I had been able, it's unlikely it would done anything for their confidence in me.

I've mentioned the heightened sense of atmosphere that can often accompany epilepsy. It's very probably this that has left it with an eerie, disturbing association, as far as many other people are concerned. For in reality, epilepsy, for most people with it, is little more than an occasional nuisance. At least, it is for me. Yet its social effects can be truly alarming and excessive. Despite its appearances, even a severe attack is almost certain to be totally painless. If there's any pain at all, it tends to come afterwards, perhaps as a result of falling or as a headache which commonly follows my more severe attacks. Otherwise, the attacks are painless, regardless of how they appear to an observer.

Other people, however, entirely understandably, tend to assume that a convulsion in particular is agonising, and do what they think will best help the person suffering it. Many, regrettably, tend to over-react to the very mention of the word, not to say an attack itself, which can provoke actual panic in others, but not in the person with the condition.

I've actually been arrested on three occasions on suspicion of drug abuse. Passers-by had mistakenly called police when in fact I was experiencing moderate seizures. I've already mentioned how it led to the collapse of my career and my marriage. For some reason, it still carries a certain, highly powerful, social disapproval.

Can epilepsy be cured? Since epilepsy is such an individual condition, that varies from person to person. Any case of the condition is subjected to a carefully planned mixture of medication (four medications in my case). If this is unsuccessful at first, alternatives are tried, possibly over a long period. Commonly, as with me, there's partial control of the condition. More than four decades after my first episodes, and a bewildering range of changing medications, I still have occasional attacks, usually for no obvious reason. It just happens.

I let these trouble me, however, as little as I possibly can, and just live a normal life, without taking senseless risks. I've learned long ago just to live with it and not let it concern me. The truly sad thing is that so many other people can't do the same, and have so often put obstacles in my way. Behaviour like theirs is something I can't make any sense of. If I don't find it a problem, most of the time, why should anyone else? For me, epilepsy isn't really a difficulty. Only one thing concerns me about it: that others may over-react to even a mild attack, something which has happened many times.

So, to describe epilepsy is anything but simple. I may not even be aware that I'm having an attack. Discovering items that I've clearly dropped on the floor, but without any knowledge of the fact, is an almost certain sign of an attack of this kind. Or there may be, say, coffee stains on a wall, yet I can't remember ever spilling a cup at those places. Or again, there may be periods, probably short, of memory loss. From time to time, I realise that I simply can't remember anything of, for example, a broadcast that I had specially marked out. Did I even hear, or see, it? I just can't say, for I've no way of knowing for sure and have to hope that it will be broadcast again.

Describing an attack of which I am aware is that it's most like what you might perhaps call a compulsory daydream. It's not very adequate, but in many years I've never hit on a better description. I don't choose then to let my attention drift off (something which I've always done from time to time in any case as a confirmed daydreamer), but instead at times it just does, confusing my senses or awareness. I can do nothing about it. There's no point in telling me, as some people have done, to

137

'pull myself together', one of the cruellest phrases in the language in my opinion. I don't deliberately have attacks, and can't just stop them.

It's important to stress, however, that there's no connection between daydreaming and epilepsy, although they may seem similar, especially to an observer. It's for this reason that schoolchildren with epilepsy are sometimes suspected of not paying attention to lessons. For them, however, it isn't a matter of choice. Yet strangely, although basic medical instruction was a compulsory part of my teacher training, this possibility wasn't mentioned. We were even instructed in noticing the first signs of leprosy, of which there hasn't been a single case in the UK in decades. But of epilepsy, there wasn't a word spoken, despite the diagnoses of thousands of cases each year. This I just can't understand.

At times, I seem to hear voices. This isn't some psychiatric disturbance, which epilepsy isn't, although that is still a common belief. It's just the result of the electrical misfires reaching the hearing area of my brain. For some time, years ago, I seemed to hear on occasion two threatening male voices. These I christened Butch and Sundance, from a favourite film of mine. Almost immediately, the voices stopped and I've never experienced them since. One of the best coping methods with epilepsy can often be humour. To worry about the condition is to give it strength, by becoming anxious. Conversely, simply laughing it off and paying it as little attention as I need to, seems to cut, so to speak, the ground from under its feet. It has nothing to fasten on to.

Very occasionally, I have a few seconds' warning of an impending attack. This is known as the epileptic aura and was first recorded in medicine at least 1,500 years ago. It's a bewildering fact that epilepsy is perhaps the longest-documented medical condition in existence, with records dating back at least to ancient Babylon, where it was thought to be caused by the Moon god, Sin. The first detailed study of the condition, still intact, in Europe was written around 400 BCE. Yet, paradoxically, it remains one of the least generally understood or accepted.

How to describe the aura? Again, it varies. Most commonly, it's a vague sense of unease, rather like when I can't remember for sure whether I've locked my door or not when going on a journey. Or it can be like a few seconds of a cold, chilling breeze (which is the original meaning of *aura*). When this does happen, I must sit down if I possibly can, grasp something firm like a chair leg (my anchor, so to speak, on reality) and concentrate on anything but epilepsy – the multiplication tables learned at school are especially useful. Even counting the number of bricks in a wall can be valuable at such times – just so long as it distracts my attention. In this way, the aura can be very useful but, at least for me, it only rarely appears, not nearly as often as even some neurologists seem to expect. This is yet another difficulty in describing the condition.

139

The success rate of this method of diverting attacks is reasonable at best. A difficulty, however, is that what seems like the aura is actually the opening stage of an attack. Nothing can be done then, for an attack will run its course and I must just recover from it. Generally speaking, that takes only a matter of minutes, if I'm left untroubled. This is the reason that public panicking can do more harm than anything else. By a ridiculous irony, I've often, even when still semi-dazed myself, had to calm down observers, who were more troubled than I was. There was even one occasion when I helped carry the stretcher of someone, a first aid officer, who felt unwell after seeing me experience an attack. That's another memory I still find always amuses me. For irony seems to be epilepsy's other name. And its worst enemy can often be humour. It's nothing to be depressed about.

Something never to do is to live in fear of it, a mistake I've never made. It's a simple fact with epilepsy that it's possible, especially with TLE, that almost anything can happen at almost any time, but that it probably won't. If we're speaking of a medical condition, as we are, those are surely good odds. In my opinion at least, I'd sooner have epilepsy than lose, say, an arm or a leg. These are difficulties which maimed people must always cope with. With most cases of epilepsy, however, there's difficulty only from time to time, sometimes more often, sometimes less. It pays to be ready for them, but not to be obsessed with them. In some countries, by comparison, I've experienced earthquakes, but returned nevertheless at later times. There was more to these places than occasional earth tremors. For most of the time, the ground stayed stable as I knew it was much more likely to do, just like anywhere else. And it's just this attitude that I take to epilepsy also – that my life is far more than it is. I have more to live for, and it won't be permitted to dominate me. It's as blunt as that.

B: FITTING IN SOCIETY

As regards this so-called 'sacred disease', these are the facts: it is no more 'sacred' or 'supernatural' than any other, but has a perfectly natural basis and normal prognosis. If I were to consider this condition 'sacred', then I might just as well say the same of innumerable conditions, such as fevers, sleep-walking and night panics.

These are some very wise words indeed. Either all medical conditions have some supernatural aspect or none has, preferably the latter. It's sobering to think that they're also the earliest words known in Europe dealing with epilepsy, the opening remarks of a short treatise on the subject, dating most probably to around 400 BCE. The author of this work, who actually uses the word epilepsy, was speaking in wry terms of what was known in his day as the 'sacred disease'. His name is uncertain. Whoever he may have been, he had the insight to attack the superstition and supposed magical treatments attached to the condition in his day.

From observation and what surely amounts to a flash of genius for his time, he correctly traced its cause to short-lived upsets in the brain, rather than to evil spirits. These had no place in his way of thinking. In saying what he did, he completely broke with the thinking of his time. It's these short disturbances that the modern EEG identifies, marking them on the graph as the characteristic 'spikes'.

It's strange, and sad, that epilepsy, possibly the longest-recorded medical condition over millennia, is still so little generally understood even in modern times. Its only real rival in those stakes is, perhaps, leprosy, a far more serious condition. Throughout that time, epilepsy has been plagued, and often still is, with superstitious notions. In our earliest references, written on clay tablets, seizures were thought to be due to the influence of the Moon. This is more dangerous than it first seems, for it leads straight to the term 'lunacy'. The Romans referred to it as the 'assembly sickness', since they supposed that if anyone had an attack during a public meeting, it must surely be a sign of divine displeasure – the same view, incidentally, as was taken of a sudden flash of lightning or roll of thunder. The meeting would be cancelled and postponed to a future, supposedly more favourable date.

Oddly, one person who had the condition himself, Julius Caesar, regularly addressed public and military assemblies, but despite the virulent political enmity common at the time there's no evidence to show that he ever had attacks at these gatherings.

Regrettably, the early author's rational attitude wasn't to spread widely or last long. By the time of the New Testament, five hundred years later, the only answer to clearly identifiable epilepsy was thought to be exorcism, to drive out the 'unclean spirit'. There was a long tradition in the more remote Scottish islands of placing a woollen net over a young baby's cradle so as, the parents hoped, to fend off future epilepsy.

This was plainly just another of the whole range of superstitions surrounding the condition. Or was it just possibly something more than that? It has been suggested, and there does actually seem to be something near the truth of the matter here. Did this practice in some way point to a subconscious sense of the brain's neural pathways, the hugely complicated network of natural 'cables' constantly carrying and transferring the brain's natural electricity? It's tempting to think so, but who can say?

Even in Martin Luther's day (mid-Renaissance), the condition was commonly known as the 'devil's disease'. As the fear of witchcraft spread over Europe, this was a dangerous notion. Why was one person affected by the condition, but not another? Had that person been perhaps collaborating with Satan? Was this a case of demonic possession? It's been suggested that Joan of Arc's supposed visions of angelic figures were actually cases of epileptic, possibly temporal lobe, attacks. From experiences of my own, I can easily accept this as a possibility. Joan, sadly, was sent to the stake. One of the last trials for witchcraft in the western world, the notorious Salem affair which resulted in a series of executions, centred largely on the evidence, so-called, of a young girl's seizures.

These superstitious ideas have actually resurfaced in recent times. This is a deeply troubling development. There are cases on record of young children being forced to swallow salt water and being brutally beaten, supposedly to drive out the imagined epilepsy demon. It's difficult, to say the least of it, to suppose that any such maltreatment would result in improvement in a medical condition. The very reverse indeed: proper

144

medical aid would be denied at a time when it was most needed by the victim of such abuse. It's only natural that the victim wouldn't refer to unobserved seizures in the hope of avoiding further spells of abuse. And as the evidence of abuse grew, the less likely it would be that those responsible (to misuse that word for the present) for it would refer to medical authorities. We're on the path here to likely brain injury and, perhaps, avoidable death.

Even in the world's most scientifically advanced country, the United States, there are reliable reports of the growing return of exorcism. I've been a reluctant witness once of this practice, outraged yet unable to intervene. I've even had the offer of exorcism myself - and firmly refused it. If medical charts and scans can identify areas of temporary disturbances in my brain's natural electricity, I've no possible reason to look for something more sinister. Neither, as I see it, has anyone else with epilepsy. It's a startling, often disturbing and inconvenient, condition, but an entirely natural one, just as much as, say, migraine. Yet migraine, at least as far as I can find out, doesn't tend to produce such bizarre behaviour in others. It seems to be a more socially acceptable condition than epilepsy, which apparently never has been – rather, the very opposite.

Exorcism is a dangerous practice. Someone who imagines he has been exorcised or 'cleansed' of his epilepsy is reasonably likely to gain psychological comfort from the idea, and so attacks may actually stop - for a time. He may stop taking prescribed medication, perhaps as a demonstration of his faith. The brain, however, the most complex object known, will tolerate this sort of neglect for only so long. After only a short time, the attacks are almost certain to return, all the more severely for being left neglected during the period of imagined cure.

To be fair, it's hard to blame others for their sudden shock when an attack occurs in public. That's simply a natural response to any such disturbance. However, an element of superstitious unease, even dread, often still surrounds the condition. In some people's eyes even now – for I've heard it said – it's as if some supernatural force has picked out the person who has had the attack, just possibly as a form of punishment. Surprisingly frequently for the present day, I've heard just this claim of spiritual punishment made as a supposed explanation for my own attacks. To my question – punishment by what and for what offence? – I've had, however, no reply. It's as if that treatise of 400 BCE had never been written. Modern society is by no means as rational as it likes to believe.

In a more mundane way, it's even possible to be suspected of drug abuse. In the past, I've more than once found myself recovering from an attack already sitting in the police interview room. It was impossible to say who was more bewildered as I gradually came round, clearly not under the influence of anything illegal. Once the position was explained, however, we parted company in mutual good humour. I expect, for the officers, it was a welcome change from genuine crime.

For this reason, it makes sense to wear a badge or bracelet to make clear just what the real difficulty is. This won't stop people panicking, but it will inform paramedics and medical staff. It also means that there's less chance of being mistakenly arrested. Panic and public ignorance can make it appear a strange, Alice in Wonderland, condition. On occasion, still dazed and shaken by a more severe attack in public, I've found myself forced to calm onlookers down, rather than receive offers of aid myself.

The attack is over, I've tried to plead, I'll be back to normal in minutes. Usually, however, it's already too late, for someone has already used his mobile phone to call for help in a supposed emergency, invariably standing at what seems a safe distance. But safe from what? Almost invariably, the only person at risk of harm from a seizure is the person experiencing it. It's surely well known that epilepsy isn't contagious – yet even in the present day there are some who think otherwise.

I've both experienced reactions like this, and observed them. Once, while I was waiting in a bus queue, a woman standing just in front of me suddenly collapsed and began convulsive trembling. I had not only my own experience, but also training in first aid to rely on. Most important was to keep her from beating her head against the concrete pavement. To protect her, I was forced to use both my forearms. No-one answered my call for a shopping bag, a rolled-up coat, anything of the kind, to use as a temporary cushion.

Everyone present had shrunk back in a staring, wide-eyed circle. I had epilepsy myself, I called again, so knew well what to do. But still no-one approached to help. At least twenty metres away, I could see a woman, obviously shocked, stammering into her mobile phone. By the time the emergency ambulance arrived, minutes later, the young woman was sitting upright, uninjured and completely back to normal. Normal, that is, except for her cringing, tearful embarrassment at having become an unwilling centre of public attention. Exasperated, I left the scene rather than make some perhaps unwise comment in the heat of the moment.

From past experience, I knew the young woman's feelings painfully well. The others present had kept their distance rather than provide the help I needed, and warned them I needed. Perhaps worse: I had seen written on their faces less human concern and understandable shock than dread. Thousands of years had passed, and nothing had changed, at least where epilepsy was concerned. People had been obviously too afraid to help – but afraid of what? This is the world in which a person with epilepsy finds himself and has to live with: one where ancestral fear often lingers on just below the modern-day surface. It can take very little to strip that veneer away.

This has been the essential problem with epilepsy through the ages, at least two and a half millennia. It seems to swing on a pendulum between sound scientific sense and outright superstition - and not just, regrettably, in so-called 'primitive' societies. It's a situation that the person with the condition has to learn to live with, at least for the time being, but not necessarily accept. His only choice is to join with organisations and press for change and do what he can for himself to make the reality of the matter known. It's disheartening, by all means, to find long-outdated notions still widely held. He must learn, over time, at least to try to shrug these off and confront mistaken claims with the actual facts.

Convincing others of the truth of the matter can be difficult, but it can be done, if not with everyone. One priceless weapon against despair can be humour. And it must be admitted that I have experienced over time kind and friendly acceptance, for example in shops. Another weapon is determination to succeed regardless in one's chosen field. That's what I made my aim

In many cases, although certainly not all, epilepsy isn't greatly significant in medical terms. It's often quite clearly, to anyone with the condition, more of a social issue. This has long been recognised. In the treatise of 400 BCE already mentioned, there's a telling paragraph:

> *People who are familiar with their condition can have a forewarning of an onset. This is when they suddenly leave company and perhaps rush home, if they live nearby, or if not, to some empty spot where only a few people will see them collapse, and then they instantly cover their heads. They do this, however, not out of dread of some supernatural force, but out of embarrassment at their condition. However, young children will run to their parents or to some other familiar adult for fear of what is about to happen to them. They have not yet learned to feel embarrassment.*

This is a clear description of social conditioning, rather than any medical aspects of epilepsy. People, in other words, just as in those times, can even now come to feel in some way socially lessened by seizures. But there's no reason that they should feel anything of the kind, any more than they should be embarrassed by, say, an injured leg or a cut finger. Why should epileptic attacks provoke a different response? It's very significant, I believe, that the word here translated as 'embarrassment' can also be translated as 'shame'. Traces of this more negative attitude linger on well into the present day. Not so very long ago, for example, people with epilepsy were prohibited from entry into Australia, under the same rule as applied to Alsatian dogs.

Social conditioning, and let's not be in any doubt about this, can be immensely powerful. Despite the support I've had from my family and friends life-long, I still commonly find myself actually apologising to bystanders when I recover from an attack. But apologise for what, when I've done nothing wrong? I honestly can't say why I do this, but I've already blurted the words out before I realise what I'm doing. This can be nothing else than a social reflex, resulting from my awareness of society's unease at epilepsy. I'm not apologetic, for I've no reason to be, yet I find I've apologised again before I could stop myself.

To describe a personal example of this social conditioning: after my curt rejection on medical grounds, by telephone and without so much as a medical examination, from teacher training college, I contacted, still shocked and bewildered, an organisation claiming to help people with epilepsy. After a day or two, a representative of the organisation drove to our family home. I still clearly remember every detail of that meeting, it left me so appalled and resentful. I should really think of myself, she suggested, not as a swan, but more as a still ugly duckling. It would be more sensible, perhaps, to set my sights low.

I could scarcely believe what I was hearing. This was her idea of help, was it, I asked? It was only a month or two since I had graduated with a good degree and several awards. Had she herself a record to match it? No, she replied, she hadn't, nothing like it. Did she have the condition herself, I continued? My question, of course, was only rhetorical since she had arrived at our home driving her own car. She shook her head. I pressed her further: did the organisation she represented have anyone with epilepsy on its staff? Almost incredibly, the answer was 'no'. Then how would she react to advice like her own if our positions were reversed? Was she actually telling me that I should consider myself somehow a lesser being, inferior, simply because of a medical condition, one that had plainly done nothing to prevent academic success? Again there was no reply.

I can only hope that at least some of the offensiveness of her own words and the indignation that she had caused had begun to dawn on her. Perhaps, or perhaps not, for she left after a few minutes, leaving me seething with outrage and with determination: determination to prove myself at least the equal of supposedly 'normal' people. No-one should be expected to tolerate what I had just heard, and I wasn't prepared to listen to anything of the kind. I did hear later, but without confirmation, that the representative had me marked down as 'irritable'. But how else could I be expected to respond to her words, except with indignation?

That wasn't the end of the matter, as far as that organisation was concerned. Some time later, I received a letter from it suggesting that I might be considered for employment, at a minimal rate, in a workshop producing surgical footwear – if, that was, I were considered suitable for such a post. This was their suggestion for a specialist in languages. I simply disposed of the letter without replying, for in my frame of mind at the time it seemed highly inadvisable to reply in the way I felt strongly tempted. Some months later, I found for myself a short-term, successful post as an unqualified teacher and the following year entered a different education college from the one to which I had first applied, in time securing a certificate with merit.

Throughout my life I've had the firm support of my family and most friends, but not, regrettably, all. Not everyone, however, is so lucky. I've already referred to the largely fictional notion of the so-called 'epileptic personality', a term frequently used in Victorian and Edwardian times, but far less in the present day. However, I have heard it used, in the recent past. This personality is depicted as the sullen and ill-natured, isolated individual, preferring to keep his own company in some dark corner.

The truth of this is rather different from the popular imagination. In the past, such medication as actually existed for the condition often had lasting and severe side effects, including violent headaches. Add to that awareness of society's attitude to epilepsy. Until well into the 20th century, anyone with epilepsy was at risk of being classed as 'mentally defective.' No-one with such a burden to bear, I think it's fair to say, would be likely to prove a brilliant conversationalist. Powerful traces of this highly negative attitude to epilepsy remain even now, as I think I've demonstrated from personal experience.

It seems worthwhile to describe the occasion when I heard the term used, only a few years before this book was written. I had just come into a café and sat down at a vacant table (I often go to cafés. I like the sense of company around me and I have the opportunity of checking up on medication in comfort.) I realised suddenly that a middle-aged woman whom I didn't know was standing close by. She wanted to apologise, she said, for her son, who was sitting in the corner just opposite. I was bewildered. Apologise for what? I'd vaguely noticed him, a young teenager, sitting quietly some tables away, when I had ordered my coffee at the counter. We certainly hadn't spoken. What could he possibly have done to offend me?

He was so withdrawn, even sullen, the woman continued, because he had the 'epileptic personality', which she went on – essentially without any basis in fact – to describe at great length. It was only when she finally completed her description that I referred, deliberately with exaggerated calm and civility, to my own epilepsy. Her stammering, embarrassed, reaction to my revelation I would find hard to describe here. I can only hope her son overheard me. At least to a point, he might have gained some very necessary confidence since I was prepared to be perfectly open about myself.

This episode might be considered absurd at first, but that's far from the real truth of the matter. In apologising, without the slightest reason, for her son's condition, she was little short of expressing shame for him, disowning him, just another form of negative social conditioning. So early in life, he was already being branded as somehow inferior by probably the closest member of his family. I had at least the impression that he had only recently been diagnosed, so would be all the more taken aback by the news. In him, I saw something of myself so many years earlier. Thankfully, however, I had had then the unfaltering support of my entire family, as I still do.

I've said above 'almost' all of my friends - but not all. A married couple whom I've known for well over twenty years fully accept me, as does their married daughter. With their adult son, however, the picture is rather different. He informed his parents, but not me personally, that he preferred not to be in my company. Apparently the simple fact that I had epilepsy made him feel uneasy and he'd rather not be in my presence if he could avoid it. I could be insulted by this if I chose to be, but there seems to be no point in taking offence at the family as a whole. Only that one person had made such a senseless and insensitive comment.

I've long since become too used to reactions of this sort for them to concern me. But wouldn't I have had good reason be offended by his comments? If I'm to be honest, I actually am to some extent, but it seems wiser not to say so, for it would do no good. Since he found my company disagreeable because of my condition, it would plainly be difficult to discuss the matter with him in person. He had simply closed the book, so to speak, on me and classed me as unacceptable. He had nothing more to say on the matter. Could anyone genuinely not find such treatment offensive and insulting? It would be a remarkable person who didn't. But what would I gain from saying so? And how could I make my point to someone who'd rather steer clear of me?

I don't know, for I've seen no point in asking, if the passing years have produced in him a more mature, accepting attitude. The irony is that, a trained scientist, he has years of experience in treating drug addiction. Yet it would probably, and I believe rightly, be thought unreasonable of me to avoid his company because of the nature of his work. I'm confronted again by that same epilepsy enigma. I'm expected to tolerate people who are unwilling to tolerate me. If I don't, if I take a stand and reply to such comments, I'm classed as the stereotype, an aggressive or irritable 'epileptic'.

What, however, I'm not prepared to do is accept such attitudes, and I take care when I can to make that known, regardless of the consequences. This can gain me the reputation of having the proverbial chip on my shoulder. But the alternative is meekness and acceptance of insults – and that amounts to conceding inferiority. That's something I will never do, for I'm in no sense an inferior. And I treat no-one as inferior to me. This is a position in which many social minorities find themselves: the dilemma of whether or not to pretend to tolerate intolerance. I stress the word 'pretend', for I'm convinced that no-one ever really tolerates insult. There's no reason why anyone should.

Until some years ago, I helped with a website, dealing with social problems, for people with epilepsy. A number of reports reached me which I found deeply troubling, showing plain signs of persistent ignorance or worse. I've no reason to disbelieve these reports. In one, a woman in the United States reported recovering from a seizure in an airport to find herself firmly fastened to a 'gurney', ominously similar to the type used when a criminal is due for execution.

In south Scotland, another young woman found herself confined overnight, after a seizure, in a psychiatric ward, where police had brought her. She, like the woman in the airport, had been wearing clear information of her condition. Epilepsy, as should be well known to anyone in authority, is not a psychiatric condition. It's entirely physical, as anyone with training in first aid, including police officers, should know perfectly well.

The worst such case was reported from the United States also. A casual worker had developed a series of seizures in his workplace. Emergency help was called. However, despite the man's workmates' protests and advice, he was placed by police under severe restraint and given no treatment. Repeated seizures (*status epilepticus*) should always be treated as the medical emergency which they are. In this particular case, lacking medical help, the man failed to survive the experience. There was no information in the report which I received whether the police officers were disciplined for their failure to treat properly what they had been told repeatedly was a medical difficulty, something which should have been obvious in any case.

So what are the realities of life with epilepsy, a 'covert' disability, at least for most of the time? There are many practical difficulties, most not immediately, if at all, obvious to someone not affected. To begin, there's no question in many cases of gaining a driving licence, often a requirement for employment, if the attacks are at all frequent. It can be very unwise to use a conventional cooker rather than a microwave oven. Even a momentary blackout anywhere near a hotplate or a gas flame can pose serious risks. I have permanent scalding marks to my back to prove that point. We mustn't use a bath, rather than a shower, unless there's help immediately available. It's only too easy, if there's an onset, to slide under the surface of the water. Not so very many years ago, that, sadly, was the fate of a prominent athlete who himself had epilepsy. Taking precautions of this sort is, obviously, nothing but good sense.

With TLE at least, or epilepsy in general, the first signs of any even slight rise in body temperature, or any lowering of one's general health condition, should serve as a warning to stay indoors, however inconvenient that may be. Better to postpone an appointment, say, than to find oneself in an Accident and Emergency ward. Even slight fever in particular is well known to aggravate seizures. And if an attack is going to occur, it's all the better (a strange word, I realise, in this context, but it's nonetheless apt) for it to take place in a familiar, home environment. That's one great advantage of keeping a medical thermometer at home, and of learning how to use it properly. The digital type, I've found, tends to be preferable, since it has a larger display and so is easier to read.

A person with epilepsy is very unwise to work with electrical equipment and in no circumstances should operate heavy machinery. Just one fleeting blackout would be enough to leave a hand permanently crushed, or perhaps much worse still. Or there could be fatal electric shock. On one of my retraining schemes, I was actually instructed, although my condition was well known, to help with operating an industrial lithograph.

This printing equipment was almost as large as a railway engine and practically as noisy. My task, I was told, would be to apply the thick black ink to the whirling metal rollers. My outright and repeated refusal to do anything of the kind, or even to go near the machine, at first caused the instructor great annoyance, and he took care to tell me so in some detail.

Within a few minutes, however, the lithograph's endless thundering began to provoke the first stages of a seizure. The instructor realised his appalling mistake and what its consequences might have been, for both him and me, if he had succeeded in cowing me. I was sent back home for the day. I had already long since learned that any unreasonable request or order, whatever the circumstances, must be refused. If that made me seem sometimes unco-operative, then that just had and still has to be the case. I know the possible alternative just too well.

Another activity I mustn't take part in, as with other people with epilepsy, is climbing, even on a secured ladder. It would be only too easy to take a chance and find myself seriously injured, perhaps even paralysed through spinal damage. I'm lucky in having obliging neighbours who are prepared to replace worn-out light bulbs for me.

Rhythmic, flickering sound or light (this is known technically as photo-sensitivity) is well known to provoke attacks in some people with epilepsy. I can speak only for myself here, for all cases have their own characteristics. Flickering light has no effect on me unless it reaches a relatively high frequency. Yet sound frequency, for some strange reason, is a different matter.

It can take no more than the steady rhythm of my own walking to provoke an attack, but only on occasion. At the first signs of this, I must stop walking altogether

158

for some time or else vary my tread. If I do either, there's at least a fair chance that the attack will go no further. A higher frequency of sound, but only rarely a lower one, can commonly cause epilepsy to flare up. The effect of the rhythmic sound of the lithograph which I've just mentioned above provides an example of sound-provoked seizures. However, there's no general rule, except perhaps the necessity to avoid flickering light and heavy machinery. As I've said earlier, if epilepsy has a particular feature, it has to be enigma. It varies enormously from person to person. The individual person must learn his own danger signs and what to avoid.

Then we have the social costs to bear, which in their own way can prove to be at least a match for the medical problems of epilepsy. Too many people, to the present day, associate disability only with the use of a wheelchair, or a walking-stick at the very least. If a condition isn't immediately evident, it can be suspected that the person claiming to be disabled is in reality simply malingering. Despite my medical history, I've had this accusation made against me. When I've tried as hard as I have, I find this thoroughly insulting – and say so. There should be no doubt that covert disabilities can often be just as much of a problem as the more obvious forms. Yet that doubt and suspicion often still attach to them. It's partly for this reason, but more to provide medical information, that I keep an epilepsy diary. Some broadcasting media are becoming aware of this situation and making such diaries available on request so as to conduct a regional survey of the condition.

However, on occasion there's the complete opposite to cope with: the people we meet who suppose that the whole of a disabled person's life must surely hinge on the disability itself. I've met so many such people. They're all the harder to deal with since they, unlike the others I've mentioned, are so desperate to help in any way they can – sometimes whether we want it or not. By doing so, they can simply just get in the way of our personal achievements and success, or just managing our lives for ourselves. We disabled people, disabled in any way, have to learn to cope for ourselves, both practically and for our own self-esteem. Self-esteem is one of the kingpins of a disabled person's world. It has to be, to counteract others' often negative or even demeaning attitudes and actions.

My world doesn't revolve round my medical condition. Why should it? In fact, I scarcely think about it, unless it forces itself on me. Otherwise, it's somewhere far out on the periphery of my being. And that, as far as I'm concerned, is where it can stay. Others, for whatever reason, think about it more than I do, and in my life it's been others' over-reactions to my epilepsy that have almost always tended to cause difficulties.

I should distinguish such over-anxious helpers, however, from those who give genuine assistance when it's actually needed, and for that reason are all the more appreciated. In my own experience, these have been predominantly younger people. It's more common for their elders to turn away or clearly pretend not to notice when I'm in difficulty. After many years of observing this, I can't avoid the conclusion that the reason for this difference in attitudes is, again, social. The younger people haven't yet had the time to absorb prevailing attitudes. To many of their elders, however, for whatever reason, people like me are troubling.

But why do I, and others like me, trouble or disturb them? If I only knew the solution to this riddle! I have said that I don't allow my epilepsy to trouble me. I accept it, and the more I accept it, the less it happens. Many other people, however, have let it trouble them, often at my cost. Whatever else, it certainly isn't my fault, as I've actually heard suggested. Is having flu the fault of the person with flu? I've never heard anyone say so.

That I can live with epilepsy and not allow it to trouble me or stand in my way isn't to say that it hasn't had an impact on my life in many ways, many of which I prefer to push to the back of my memory, for to bring them to mind would be only to reopen wounds. There are two issues, however, that I can't treat this way. They're the pointless ruin of what might have been a fruitful career.

Worse, there's the senseless destruction of my personal family life, which I witnessed on that ghastly March day so many years ago. I wasn't allowed, I later discovered, even to remain in photographs taken in those years. How am I to forgive that level of malice? I genuinely wish that I could forgive all that happened then, but I can't. The people responsible for it are mostly by now well beyond human retribution. No, I can't forgive them, and don't see why I should be expected to. Should I forgive the malice and stupidity of people who wouldn't forgive my epilepsy, even make an effort to understand it? Besides, to forgive what happened then would be the ultimate disloyalty to the

161

person who suffered most from their actions. I can allow myself a perfectly human sense of resentment, but I know it's vital to avoid hatred.

People such as those I've just mentioned have seen my disability, a minor aspect of me, as a form of distorting mirror for the whole person. They weren't to be told differently, however hard I tried. It's an experience disabled people come to know well: that a part of us can often be treated as more important than the whole. What, however, we mustn't ourselves do is view society as a whole in the same distorted perspective. Our viewpoint must be brighter, our vision clearer, than our critics' own. For, simply by responding naturally to their own wilder claims, we can find ourselves appearing to prove them in the right.

It's a position that a number of minority groups know only too well. The more vigorously we react to offensiveness, ignorance, exclusion or worse, the more we seem to confirm the stereotype rather than weaken it. Yet we can't be expected to stay silent and pretend such things don't happen, just to seem to improve our image. That won't happen, for the truth of this was expressed long ago: silence can be taken as a sign of acceptance. This is a negative cycle that must be broken somehow. Making the true facts known may just be one way of doing so. But, as we all know, you can never make people listen.

C: THE ROAD AHEAD:
WHICH WAY NOW?

The main problem of epilepsy, I'm convinced from years of experience, is that it's shackled to its history. This is not a desirable history, far from it. Rather, it's one crammed with unfounded notions of lunacy or mental defect, criminality (the once-fashionable notion of the 'criminal profile' was formed largely from a series of photographs of people with the condition. On that ridiculous basis, people were warned to avoid anyone whose eyes were too close together or too far apart, for example), demons, evil spirits and other such hobgoblins.

None of these has any place in a modern, rational mind. To be strictly logical, if some supposed spiritual force causes seizures, does it cause, say, dandruff and bunions too? I've never heard anyone suggest so. Spiritual or natural (which includes psychological) causes: it's one or the other; it can't be both. I know which I believe makes sense. Since medication clearly reduces, sometimes eliminates, seizures, there's no space left for spirits or demons. Modern-day surgical equipment can trace the irregularities in brain electricity which give rise to seizures. Something it finds no trace of is evil spirits or anything else of the kind. It's time, then, and long has been, to break that link with the past and its superstitions.

What are the modern developments? There are many, including an advance on the EEG (electro-encephalogram), the MRI scanner (magnetic resonance imaging). This provides a highly-detailed picture of the inner areas of the brain. I've gone through this pain-free procedure on two occasions and have seen for myself the most likely cause of my own seizures. It's a bundle, about the size of a small chestnut, of redundant tissue just above and behind my right ear. Since it's a likely, but not definite, cause of the attacks, I decided against surgery and preferred to rely on medication. It's for other people to make their own choices for or against surgery when offered, for it isn't always an option. I can't make suggestions for anyone else. It has to be an individual choice, depending on qualified advice.

And what about that medication? There are many different preparations available, some in use for many years and newer substances coming into use. Some are completely successful in overcoming epilepsy, some only partly, reducing the frequency or the intensity of attacks. It's this latter group I belong to: my condition is lessened, but not completely eradicated. I'm content with that. I've learned to live with epilepsy and don't let it trouble me or stand in my way. I've used it as a launch pad, not a brick wall. What I certainly don't do is worry about it. I take reasonable precautions, take medication as prescribed and that's all there is to it.

There's a particularly sensible reason for not worrying about it. Worry is a form of stress, and stress is a particularly effective trigger of seizures. If

I did worry, I'd be a threat to myself. That alone is one good reason for thinking about it as little as I do. In any case, I've too much else to occupy my time.

There's no one-for-all treatment for epilepsy. Each case has to be assessed individually, and one or more types of medication tried over what can be a considerable time. In my case, I rely on a mixture of four medications, reaching well over 4,000 milligrams a day. Carrying supplies with me, especially if I'm away from home for any length of time, can be inconvenient. However, I know the alternative.

A standard rule, not only with epilepsy, is that any medication has side-effects of some sort. A change of medication is likely to have unfamiliar, perhaps undesirable, effects. If these last more than a reasonable time or are clearly excessive, they should be reported as soon as possible. It seems likely that this is either the wrong dosage, or the wrong medication,. One thing that always is well worth checking is the manufacturer's insert. Perhaps what you're experiencing isn't unusual at all, has been widely reported, and can be counted on to wear off in no great time.

You could reasonably say, I believe, that epilepsy has three problems, all with the initial 'S'. They're superstition, stereotype and stigma. Superstition I've already dealt with: it's a collection, nothing more than that, of completely baseless and outdated fears, dating back in some cases to before recorded history. What do you do with people who hold these ideas? If they insist on ignoring evidence that disproves their fears, and many do, there's not much you can do for them. They're the losers where this issue is concerned. A person with epilepsy who is clear about the facts of his condition has the upper hand. His side of the story can be proved; superstition never can be.

Now for the stereotype: the disabled person (and here I'm referring not only to epilepsy) is still too often portrayed as some hopeless, helpless inferior hoping for a few coins to come his way. That's totally wrong. Over the years, I've come to see disability as hardly a medical issue at all, but a social one. It's what other people think the disabled person can't do, instead of what the disabled person knows he can do. It's more society and its attitudes that disable someone than a medical condition itself. The answer to that is obvious: prove it wrong.

This is why I believe it's vital for any disabled person to achieve everything he's capable of, and then try something more. Every time that a disabled person achieves something, the stereotype is shaken just that little bit more. I've given my own history. Probably I overdid things time and again, but I'm all the more pleased about that. I'd willingly do it all over again.

I've deliberately held the gaze of interviewers who rejected me on grounds of 'over-qualification'. So I'd managed more, I gradually made a point of asking, than able-bodied potential colleagues? Then how could I be called disabled? Often that question caused embarrassment. It was meant to do just that. I wanted them to realise that they just weren't talking sense. It's more than a little significant, I think, that none ever answered the killer question: how could I be at the same time both 'too able' and yet not able enough?

Disability – and this point can't be stressed often enough or hard enough – isn't the same as inability. The two words may certainly look or sound similar, but that's as far as it goes. Probably the finest physicist in Britain, perhaps worldwide, is Professor Steven Hawking, himself gravely disabled, if not with epilepsy. There are many other examples of achievement in the teeth of supposed incapacity or supposedly diminished ability.

But for the moment, we'll stick with epilepsy. If someone has an ability or capacity, he should go straight ahead and put it to good use, epilepsy or no epilepsy. Unless the condition has an obvious bearing on that ability, it should just be ignored. Even if it does have a bearing, there's usually some other angle to exploit the ability without taking unreasonable risks.

Very often, there are nothing like as many risks as other people care to imagine. This is the reason that, in writing this book, I've not kept my usual rule, to make little of my own achievements in a range of areas over the years. I refused to let people stop me doing what I knew I could do – and I was proved to be in the right, as my list of certificates and awards demonstrates. It's easily possible to be virtually strangled with over-protection. The answer to that is to force it aside regardless. It's the person with the condition who knows for himself what he can or can't do, and what his own limits are.

In just this way, people with epilepsy have done much for humanity over the centuries. We know for a fact, as I've said, that Julius Caesar had some form of epilepsy. That didn't prevent him from becoming probably the finest military tactician of his day and a first-rate politician who did much to reform the Roman law code. His own expertly-written and detailed reports survive to the present day. He was aware, unlike many others, that the calendar of his time was becoming outdated and falling out of synchrony with the seasons. This, he knew, just wasn't his skill, but he knew where to find someone who could be relied on to correct it. This is partly why the calendar we still use has the month of July, in his honour, named after him.

There's the artist Van Gogh, whose colour work undeniably owes much to the colour distortions experienced in his TLE. I recognised this immediately I first saw his paintings. I've no doubt he used his seizures in a positive, practical way. There's other art work where I've noticed some oddly familiar use of colour and dimensions. However, I've never found definite evidence of epilepsy in the life stories of those artists. Perhaps, in some instances, it was concealed as somehow shameful. Given, nonetheless, that so many people have the condition, it only stands to reason that I must be correct in at least some of my suspicions.

Then there's the area of literature. Authors known to have had epilepsy include Edgar Allan Poe in the USA; in France we have Guy de Maupassant, a fine author of short stories in particular, and Flaubert. These often show a touch of the strange and mysterious, for example Poe's *Masque of The Red Death* or *The Fall of The House of Usher*. I'm convinced, from my own experiences, that I see the influence here of epileptic hallucinations.

Without doubt the most positive literary figure where epilepsy is concerned is the 19th Century Russian author Dostoyevsky. It's a matter of record that he regarded his seizures, mainly the first signs of onset, as little short of a blessing. They seem to have provided him, at least in his view, with the basics of a story or a chapter of a book. It is true that a number of his works do feature characters with epilepsy, for example in *The Brothers Karamazov*. There's some evidence that the composer Tchaikovsky showed signs of a condition that may possibly have been a form of epilepsy. However, the evidence we have is nowhere near enough to be convincing. It's at least possible.

Regarding epilepsy as a near-blessing is perhaps an over-reaction, but at least a positive one. Yet in Britain, all of the figures I've just named would, not long ago, be treated as virtually insane. The society they contributed to would have rejected and excluded them

In our own day, we have the British author, historian of religion and documentary film maker, Karen Armstrong. A description of her own experiences of epilepsy, discrimination, yet eventual success, is best found in her short work, *The Spiral Staircase* (2004). Much of what she describes is painfully familiar to me personally, and no doubt to many others. I wanted to contribute far more than I actually did, but for a range of half-baked misconceptions was actively prevented from doing so.

People with epilepsy have given much to society over many centuries, sometimes actually inspired, as I've shown, by their condition. Too often, and even now, their reward has been rejection. This is something I've often considered over the years. Why, even when faced with evidence of ability, has society so often chosen to turn its face away, even when accepting other conditions albeit sometimes reluctantly? I sincerely wish I could reach any other conclusion to this riddle, but I can't. It has to be that we're confronting the remaining vestiges of atavistic superstition.

The reappearance of supposed exorcism even in advanced societies makes that point painfully plain. We can only wonder what that unnamed physician of 2,400 years ago, whose acid comments I translated in the previous section, would make of the position now. He'd surely shake his head in disbelief that so little has changed. Much of what he wrote on the matter is still readily recognisable in society today.

We have to be careful, too, to avoid a sentimental notion: that disabled people who achieve do what they do *because* they're disabled, that nature conferred on them a special gift to compensate for their problems. Nature isn't as kindly as that. If there's any truth in this notion at all, it's more this: that a disabled person will concentrate all the more on some ability that he does have in any case. He does this to compensate for what others perceive him as being unable to do. I'm speaking from my own experience, for it's what I myself did, and still do. I still translate, if only for my own interest. We try extra hard to prove ourselves, for we have to, just to prove others' misconceptions wrong and, more importantly, to reach our full potential for our own satisfaction. We have to take a pride in ourselves, no less than anyone else.

Perhaps the biggest problem to be faced is this: how do you counteract stigma? Stigma can be painful, for more than the disabled person. It destroyed my own family life. Intimate relationships involving disabled people can often be frowned on, sometimes condemned outright. That's not confined to so-called 'developing' countries. I've heard it in Britain also, in recent times.

Until no great time ago, even in some of the states of North America, marriage was actually prohibited for people with epilepsy. In other countries, sterilisation has at times been compulsory. Yet there's only limited evidence that epilepsy is hereditary, at all frequently. And even if it were, would it be really so terrible for people with epilepsy to marry anyway? If it comes to that, an epilepsy-free family, with no past history of the condition, can suddenly find itself with an idiopathic case, completely without explanation. Precisely that happened in my own family's case one November night. They, to their credit, were prepared to support me.

In many cases, however, people with the condition can still find themselves rejected, even by their own families. There's only one consideration

171

to keep in mind. A potential partner in any relationship should be aware of the other partner's condition and be prepared to accept it. Apart from that, the matter is no-one else's to interfere with.

When epilepsy is the result of injury or illness, it's obviously impossible for the condition to be inherited. One objection made is that no-one who has difficulties with employment should have children to keep. There's a simple solution to what isn't a genuine problem: employment should be made easier to gain and keep, regardless of epilepsy, free of senseless discrimination. We can have much to offer, as I've tried to show - when we're allowed to do so. Yet, too often, we're not.

A few years before writing this book, I was wondering about just this. At the time, I was walking through a street market. It struck me: isn't stigma a sign of what nobody's prepared to mention? I found myself wondering, why, when epilepsy is as common as it is, do we so rarely hear the word mentioned? Bookshops increasingly bristle with help-yourself guides to a range of often more obscure, far rarer, conditions. But any dealing with epilepsy have been difficult to come by, except on-line. But this has been the characteristic of a number of liberalisation movements over recent years: someone, each time, spoke the unspeakable word. Was epilepsy, then, the unspeakable condition? Not as far as I was concerned, not any longer. I was going to do more than just speak it, whether or not anyone else would.

In the street market, there was a badge maker's stall. I admit to a twinge of nervousness, a lasting effect of social conditioning, as I went up to him and gave him my order. An hour or so, and a cup of coffee later, my order was ready. It was a lapel badge bearing the words: Fit For Life With Epilepsy (the ambiguity of 'fit' was, of course, deliberate).

Why do this? It was simple enough. I was determined to speak the unspeakable word. Either I could cower in a corner somewhere or adopt the 'in your face' attitude – and that was just what was needed. The badge said: this is the person I am, and this is the condition I have. You can take me or leave me. And I'll do the same with you, depending on your reaction to me. No, this wasn't aggressive. It was, and still is, both assertive and informative. With epilepsy, I needed to be both.

What's happened in the years since has both surprised and gratified me. I've had only a single negative, hostile reaction, and that was from someone who wasn't sober, someone in other words who was responsible for the state he was in. I'm not. Certainly, there have been many people, shop assistants etc, who have shown surprise at first, but only for seconds. They were startled, I'm convinced, that someone was prepared to stand up and say the word – referring to himself.

I believe it's even done some good in other ways. In a shop, I could just hear two elderly women talking about the badge, with the name of evidently a young boy audible. I can only assume they were speaking about some young relative with the condition. Perhaps seeing me going around in a perfectly natural way, doing everyday things,

173

heartened them. I hope that's the case – and if it is I'm delighted. On a few occasions I've actually been approached by strangers who referred to the badge and asked for advice on how to deal with the condition in a relative. My advice has always been: to make as little of it as possible. It's what I've done.

And that, just possibly, could be the key to a beginning of a solution to the social problems caused by epilepsy. The word has to be said more often, not skirted round as I've heard even some physicians do. The more it's said, the more common the condition is realised to be. Better still: the more often the word is said, the less power it has to cause alarm, for it becomes something familiar, no longer something eerie or strange, or unacceptable. I can hope, and I certainly believe, the more it's mentioned, the more other people will understand it. If I openly show the word applies to me, then, for me, there can't be stigma. If I'm not troubled by it, no-one else surely should be.

There's an enormously important point: that the person with epilepsy shouldn't allow himself to become isolated, but mix socially whenever possible. Ideally, that should be in person, but now it doesn't need to be, when that's impracticable for some reason, say if someone lives in an outlying area. Another way of extending one's social circle is through the keyboard. This way, it becomes possible to chat on-line with people almost anywhere world-wide. This can deal with discussing the effects of epilepsy itself, and so finding how many others there are like you, that you're far from alone, and how the matter's dealt with in various other parts of the world. Or there can be a sharing of practically any other interests. Contact of this kind, I've found, can lead before long to actual personal contact.

Just to take a single example: I've had a good friend for a number of years, but have never met him since we're separated by 5,000 miles of the Atlantic Ocean. He set up a web-site for people with epilepsy and, for some years, I contributed many articles to it. Most of the many readers, though not all, were in the United States and Canada. In a strange way, I still feel a sort of association with them. It's heart-warming to think that there's possibly some help my articles have provided. And all this took was tapping at a keyboard.

So, for the many, many people with epilepsy, what's the future to be? I believe it depends on us to a large extent. We must be prepared to say the word, without shame or embarrassment. The more the word's spoken, the wider information and knowledge gradually spread. It's slow but it happens, and we have to make it happen. I made a start by wearing my badge. Yet I can scarcely manage single-handed. Badges don't cost much. All it takes is to pluck up the courage to have one made, and wear it prominently. That's how widespread under-standing often begins – with what seems like little more than a gesture.

Michael Igoe
July 2008

SUGGESTED FURTHER READING

<u>Introduction</u>: Despite many years' personal experience of epilepsy and its consequences, I still prefer not to include a list of even the most basic terms associated with it, in the sketchiest of detail. The reason for my decision is simple enough. As I commented at the outset of this book, my intention is to deal with the social aspects of epilepsy, based on my own life experience. I have no medical background, only that experience. Neurology in particular is vastly too complex for me even to attempt a glossary.

There is one word, however, which I do want to deal with here: 'epileptic'. It's never correct to use this of a person with epilepsy. If anything, I consider it demeaning, even when a doctor uses it of me, as I've known to happen occasionally. I'm not 'an epileptic', and neither is anyone else with the condition. This word can certainly be used, of the condition itself and its symptoms (e.g. 'epileptic fit' etc.), but not of the person himself, or herself. It just so happens that I'm a person with epilepsy, and have been for many years. What I'm not, however, is 'an epileptic', and I never have been.

This isn't an exercise in that weary, over-used term, 'political correctness', which I consider almost meaningless. It's a far more practical and important consideration. If the word is used of a person, it amounts to hanging a label round his neck. And it's a label many people, even now, consider objectionable, as I know to my cost. It's seen by them for some reason as the most important aspect of that person, not what he has to offer his society or his employer – and, therefore, to his family. In other words, to use the word in this way is to stigmatise him. So, throughout this book, I've referred to 'people with epilepsy', not 'epileptics'. 'Epileptics' don't exist, at least as far as I'm concerned. And I hold the same opinion of other medical conditions also. In my personal opinion, there are no 'schizophrenics', 'diabetics' or 'alcoholics'. These are people with schizophrenia, diabetes or alcoholism. The person must come first, and the condition after. We aren't medical files with a name attached, but persons with a particular medical problem, epilepsy or whatever else. We don't refer to the average person, prone to flu, as 'an influenzic'. So why refer to someone as 'an epileptic'? There's much more to him or her than that. It's only a tiny part of a person with much to offer.

Titles on the subject of epilepsy can be surprisingly difficult to find on the shelves of bookshops – surprising when epilepsy is as common as it is. For that reason, most of the books I've listed below have to be specially ordered, or bought on-line.

It's wise to use the internet with great care, on anything referring to medical conditions. A distinguished specialist in the care of epilepsy has expressed great alarm at the inaccuracies in much of what he's found on the net, some of it potentially actually harmful. It's highly important to check any information with a qualified medical professional or a recognised organization. Where, however, the internet is enormously valuable is in preventing epilepsy from being the isolating condition that it has been for many years. Internet groups, for simply chatting and sharing experiences, not just about epilepsy, can be contacted worldwide, so that the illusion that the person diagnosed is practically alone on Earth – an easy impression to gain – isn't long in disappearing.

From diagnosis onwards, it only makes sense to be crystal-clear about everything you're told about the condition. If you're not told, be sure to ask, in as much detail as you can. But there's a part you can play too. That's in providing details of onsets. Medical professionals have to rely on information provided, which is what only the person with the condition, or an observer, can do. If both can give information, that's even better. A seizure of any kind can certainly be dispiriting and exhausting, which can make putting pen to paper an unattractive prospect at first. Just a few early outline notes will be enough, and these can be written up in more detail later. These notes can be used also to record any side-effects of prescribed medication. Information of this kind is enormously valuable too. The information which I've collected on my own attacks in just this way has been borrowed by hospitals near my home, and I still make sure to provide regular copies of my notes. It's only this type of first-hand information which makes proper treatment of any case of epilepsy at all possible. And

179

without this type of information, none of the following books could ever have been written.

Orrin Devinsky M.D: *Epilepsy, Patient and Family Guide* (various editions, F.A. Davis). This is, in my personal opinion, the most useful and informative book on epilepsy available at present to the general reader. The author is, among other posts held, Director of the Comprehensive Medical Centre, New York University. He takes great care in explaining in detail the various forms of epilepsy, medication available, and not only the necessary limitations imposed by the condition, but also the many remaining possibilities in life, which it needn't affect at all. Naturally, it deals with the subject from an American perspective, but this has little effect on the quality of advice given to people with the condition, and their families, world-wide. A medical condition isn't, of course, concerned with nationality.

Brian Chappell and Dr Pamela Crawford: *Epilepsy At Your Fingertips* (Class Publishing, London). The joint authors have much close experience with epilepsy, Mr Chappell having worked with the British Epilepsy Association, and Dr Crawford a consultant neurologist. This is a very handy practical guide, similar to Devinsky but on a rather smaller scale. Its advantage, of course, since it is a British work, is that sees epilepsy and its various treatments from the perspective of the United Kingdom, many of whose institutions have close parallels in the British Commonwealth.

EPILEPSY ORGANISATIONS

In the internet age, there's no real limit to contact with organisations practically world-wide. There can be a lot to gain simply by looking into the web-sites of other countries' organisations and by investigating attitudes to epilepsy there. Not only that; it's easily possible to make contact with individual people overseas who have the condition themselves, and share experiences and views with them, and not necessarily just on your medical condition, but life and interests generally. I've done just that for a number of years with someone else with TLE in New York, but without ever meeting him in the flesh. His input into the effects of a particular medication was invaluable to me. Even inland, it makes a lot of sense to get in touch with organisations which possibly aren't active in your particular area, but can still provide information. Information is the key to living with epilepsy, and yet, for some reason, it's often sadly lacking. For this reason, the person diagnosed with the condition can feel very isolated and alone. The truth of the matter is very different. It's estimated that, world-wide, around forty to fifty million people have the condition in some form or other. A number of these organisations have chat rooms for conversation. The introduction of video messaging in particular means that you might as well be sharing a room with your on-line companion, who may in reality be thousands of miles away. Making contact in this way, inland or overseas, is well worth the little effort involved. Since this is a universal issue, only a few can be listed here. An internet search will bring many more to light.

UK Organisations

Epilepsy Research (previously The Fund for Epilepsy): A particularly active group, originally based in Halifax, Northern England, but now in London. Contact details: P.O. Box 3004, London W4 4XT, tel. 020 8995 4781, www.epilepsyresearch.org.uk

Epilepsy Action: runs a valuable chat-group, forum. Like the organizations listed below, one of the major groups concerned with the condition in the UK. New Anstey House, Gate Way Drive, Yeadon, Leeds LS19 7XY, tel. 0113 2108800, www.epilepsy.org.uk

National Society for Epilepsy: Chalfont Centre for Epilepsy, Chalfont St Peter, Bucks SL9 0RJ, tel. 01494 601 300, www.epilepsynse.org.uk

Epilepsy Scotland: 48, Govan Rd, Glasgow, G51 1JL, tel. 0141 427 4911, epilepsyscotland.org.uk

Epilepsy Connections: Active mainly in Southern Scotland, based in Glasgow, but easily contacted by internet for information: 100, Wellington St, Glasgow G2 6DH, info@epilepsyconnections.org.uk.

The Muir Maxwell Trust: contact www.muirmaxwelltrust.com (based in Edinburgh).

The National Centre for Young People With Epilepsy (NCYPE): St Piers Lane, Lingfield, Surrey RH7 6PW, tel. 01342 32243, www.ncype.org.uk

Irish Republic

Brainwave, 249, Crumlin Rd, Dublin 12, Ireland, tel. 00 3531 455 7500 (from UK), www.brainwave@iol.ie.

USA

Mainly The Epilepsy Foundation of America: 4351, Garden City Drive, Landover, MD 20785, tel. (800) 332-1000 or (301) 459-3700, www.efa.org or www.epilepsyfoundation.org. This large organisation runs a particularly active web-site and is especially handy for making overseas contacts.

International League Against Epilepsy: www.ILAE.org, A range of chapters and regions. Not by any means the organisation only for professionals as it may first appear. Its range of aims, resources, and accomplishments is well worth investigation by anyone connected in any way with the condition.